T0246015

Praise for *Danny's People*

'A beautifully written and wonderful insight into the challenges, and yes, the rewards of autism. We all need to read this book and be inspired by its uplifting message.'

Jon Snow

'Moving and deeply thoughtful, Virginia Bovell writes about happiness and struggle with an evenly light touch. She has managed to entwine politics and heart, theory and lived experience so simply and seamlessly that each seems inseparable from the other. At last!'

Sally Phillips

'Virginia's love for her son Danny is an inspiring testament and a celebration of neurodiversity. This important book dismantles prejudice and shines with honesty and truth.'

Manni Coe, author of *Brother. Do. You. Love. Me.*

'A remarkable book that raises deep questions. Her [Virginia's] compassion for autistic people – in all their multiplicity – and the dedicated people who support them shines through. This book will inspire and educate.'

Prof Simon Baron-Cohen, Director of the
Autism Research Centre, University of Cambridge

'A book of fierce compassion, wisdom and love – inspirational.'

Dr Gavin Francis, author of *Adventures in Human Being*

'An impassioned plea for better provision for autistic people, as well as a moving and unsparing account of the joys and challenges of raising Bovell's autistic son… *Danny's People* radiates with love and Bovell's warm voice.'

Jill Dawson, author *The Great Lover*

'Virginia and I first met when we took on the mammoth task of setting up a school for autistic children in the late 90s. *Danny's*

People is both a rollercoaster of emotion and a wonderful resource. It confronts a question that haunts parents like Virginia and me: who will look after our children when we're no longer around?'
Dr Anna Kennedy OBE, author of *Not Stupid*

'A beautifully written and searingly honest account of the highs and lows of raising a disabled child... a must-read for anyone who would benefit from a critical and empathetic reflection on a range of debates and controversies in the field of autism.'
Professor Laura Crane, Director of The Autism Centre for Education and Research at the University of Birmingham

'Virginia Bovell's marvellous book goes to the heart of what it takes to parent a profoundly disabled young man. It charts with tremendous care and unflinching honesty the fearfully challenging health complications faced by her beloved son, Danny, but also the radiant joy that he inspires in so many... *Danny's People* is an important, honest and beautiful book.'
Stephen Unwin, director and former chair of Kids

'A profound, insightful and deeply moving book, *Danny's People* explores the human relationships that lie at the very core of any thriving life... The result is not just one of the best recent contributions to autism research, but one of the most compelling books that I have read in many years.'
Liz Pellicano, Professor of Autism Research, UCL

'Virginia's humanity, warmth and dedication to doing whatever she can to help those who are marginalised and particularly those with learning difficulties or who get the label of autism, shine through. Her son Danny's life and experience leaps out of the pages, helping the reader see into the uniqueness of the world he inhabits and beyond the superficiality of sympathy and stereotypes.'
Dr Sami Timimi, author of *The Myth of Autism*

Danny's People

A Memoir and Manifesto
About Autism

VIRGINIA BOVELL

ONEWORLD

A Oneworld Book

First published by Oneworld Publications Ltd in 2024

ISBN 978-0-86154-838-5
eISBN 978-0-86154-839-2

Typeset by Geethik Technologies
Printed and bound in Great Britain by Clays Ltd, Elcograf S.p.A.

Oneworld Publications Ltd
10 Bloomsbury Street
London WC1B 3SR
England

Stay up to date with the latest books,
special offers, and exclusive content from
Oneworld with our newsletter

Sign up on our website
oneworld-publications.com

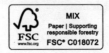

Contents

Author's Note   vii
Prologue   ix

PART 1   NEW LIFE   1
1   Danny   5
2   An Introduction to Autism   13
3   No Man's Land   18
4   Kidzmania   23
5   On the Margins   27
6   Sarah, and the Challenge of Inclusion   33

PART 2   CONNECTIONS AND CAMPAIGNS   37
7   Early Intervention   41
8   ABA: Good News?   45
9   ABA: The Controversy   50
10 TreeHouse   55
11 Su and Elliot   59
12 Marching   62

PART 3   SOLIDARITY AND CONFLICT   67
13 Donna, Daniel and Paul   71
14 The MMR Controversy   75
15 MMR and Simon Murch   81
16 Corey   87
17 Four Prayers   92
18 Depression and Identity   96
19 Debbie   104
20 Reflections   112

PART 4   THE WHIRLWIND YEARS, 2006–9   117
21 John   121
22 Larry, and the Wider Autism Movement   123
23 Tribalism   130
24 ABA Tribes and Michelle Dawson   136
25 Arsenal and Arsène Wenger   145
26 The Queen   149
27 Dinah   151
28 The Wrights and Rights   157
29 Groundhog Years   163
30 Lee   169

PART 5   THE BIG QUESTIONS   177
31 Helen Keeler and Eugenics   181
32 Ingrid   187
33 Light and Shadow   191
34 Home and Away   196
35 Surgery   202
36 Spring and Summer 2013   209
37 Crisis   213

PART 6   UNCERTAINTY AND BELIEF   229
38 Disagreements and the Empathy Question   233
39 The Future of Autism   239
40 Valuing Learning Disability   247
41 How Things are Now   252

Notes   261
Select Bibliography   285
Acknowledgements   305

Author's note

'How can I find my people? [...] I'd like to
find my "tribe".'

Adult recently diagnosed with
autism spectrum disorder, *Quora*

This is the story of my son Danny and me, and the people and
ideas we have encountered on our journey. Our story is personal
of course, but it connects with the lives of others who have
been impacted by autism and disability more generally, not to
mention fundamental questions of individual and group identity. Many people have strong feelings and beliefs in these areas,
and I have had to confront my own. In so doing I have struggled to reconcile what often appear to be opposing standpoints
and allegiances. This book emerged from the crucible of that
struggle.

PROLOGUE

When I was an undergraduate, I found myself with friends standing in a freezing-cold shopping centre, wet with snow and sleet, seeking signatures for a Spastics Society (as it was then titled) petition requesting improved services for disabled people. A young woman from the charity had come to speak about the campaign and to ask for volunteers, so my friends and I donned scarves, gloves and clipboards and braved the elements.

It was remarkably easy to elicit signatures. I do not think this was just because we were a pitiful sight in the cold, teeth chattering as we explained the cause. What struck me forcefully about that freezing morning was how many people told me that they had a relative or a friend with a disability. They were eager to sign and wanted to share their stories. The message came over loud and clear that disabled people are ubiquitous – but invisible.

Outside of the mainstream world, on the fringes, they may be everywhere, but they – or their impairments – are hidden from public view and, thus, mainstream consciousness. That same shopping centre in midsummer would appear no less devoid of disabled people than it was on that snowy morning. Wherever I went, to lectures, to parties, to clubs, on trains and buses, just going about life, I met virtually no disabled people. I had no disabled friends. If I had examined my assumptions, I would have encountered the patronising view that the disabled were a poor unfortunate minority languishing somewhere indoors, in families of people I did not know or in care homes and hospitals I had never visited. They were a tragic minority to be pitied, living as if on the other side of the world.

And yet, the lessons of that morning stayed with me: the surprise of learning that disability runs throughout the fabric of our species and that the full story of the world we live in extends way beyond what we see and hear upfront. There were barriers preventing disabled people from coming into full view and − I would later learn − such barriers included environmental and attitudinal obstacles that were quite separate from any impairment that an individual might have.

Despite this glimmer of awareness, a question I did not ask myself was this: was it a political act, to seek signatures for the petition, or was it an act of compassion, perhaps, for some, of condescension? Only many years later would this question become central to my life.

As the mother of a disabled child, my campaigning activity initially focused on the traditional arenas of politics in the UK − holding meetings with government ministers, MPs and senior civil servants, organising fringe events at party conferences, lobbying professional bodies and talking to journalists. It would take far longer for the issues of power, status and identity to find their way into my home, my life and my very sense of who I am and who my son is. My impression of what it is to be a thriving human versus an inadequate human, of being someone who is ill versus someone who merely fails to conform to wider societal expectations. I would need to hear from different people, read their accounts and meet them.

And after that, I would need to tell Danny's story.

Part 1

NEW LIFE

'There's not just love in this story, but luck. There is both bright luck and dark luck. [...] Dark luck is not bad luck. Luck can be shrouded and half-shadowed, if its outcome takes years – even half a lifetime – to be revealed.'

Riva Lehrer, *Golem Girl*

Many of us create narratives about our lives, and in writing about my own I am no exception. Yet I do not know how – or even if – Danny goes through a similar process of recall and reflection. If I were to ask him about this, I believe that he would not understand the question, let alone articulate a response. Nor can he give informed consent to being written about (unlike the other people in this book).

But I have persisted, for better or worse.

I hope that, were he to comprehend the content of these pages, Danny would forgive me for any misjudgement or intrusions into his privacy. I hope he would be pleased to share with you the surprises and discoveries, the sheer good luck that has prevailed over the setbacks, and the love that continues to carry us forward.

1

DANNY

The story starts in the spring of 1993. I am pregnant for the first time, and here sit Nick and I, just married, at our first antenatal meeting.

We had met seven years earlier. At that time Nick was a struggling writer, scraping a living as a part-time teacher in an English language school. He introduced me to Arsenal Football Club and new kinds of music, books and films. He was funny and clever and patient with my restlessness, as I worked my way through several attempts at a career: nurse, health visitor, health promoter, health economist and, finally, social policy researcher at the London School of Economics.

Now – having weathered various storms, and just at the point when Nick's first book, *Fever Pitch*, has been shortlisted for the prestigious NCR prize for non-fiction – we are expecting our first baby. The scene is set for a new life, a new chance for us, new friendships, new futures. And so here we are, introducing ourselves to the other couples.

All first children represent a turning point in the lives of their parents, and the first antenatal class is a kind of landmark. But as I return to the scene, what stands out is the significance of meeting Ingrid and her partner Hugh.

Ingrid and Hugh were instantly likable. Both were tall and striking, benign, self-deprecating and gently humorous. Immediate connections were reflected in later discoveries: Hugh and I were both from Sussex, and we found out that he went to school with childhood friends of mine. Ingrid, in contrast, had come to England from South Africa, to escape apartheid and to continue the struggle by working in immigration law. We were two couples in love, full of hope for our babies and our relationships, and – as luck would have it – living within five minutes' walk of one another in Highbury, the home of Arsenal Football Club.

★

Ingrid and I went into labour on the same day and stayed on the same ward at Homerton Hospital. Ingrid delivered Jack first. Danny took longer – he got stuck, and I had a fainting episode which was treated as a fit, so I, and therefore Danny, was pumped full of anticonvulsants. The epidural sent my blood pressure falling inexorably downwards. I began to see double and the medics around me sounded worried. I wondered if I would die and, without panic but with a good deal of regret, lamented the possibility that I'd never know what would happen to these beloved people – Nick and our baby.

But I was very much alive and awake for the emergency Caesarean, with Nick at my side. After the preceding drama, the procedure felt surprisingly relaxed. There was chat about football (our anaesthetist was an Everton supporter), what name we might give our baby and how much we loved the NHS.

And now here he is, our little Danny, perfect in my arms and feeding from my breast. Sweet and beautiful and beloved.

When we left hospital it was raining and it continued to rain for what felt like months and months. But it was only rain. Nick would write of the happy time of Danny's early days and weeks, and I was one of the lucky ones who, despite being physically depleted and exhausted, did not fall prey to the ravages of post-natal depression.

'It's like falling in love,' I explained to a friend. I hope I didn't sound smug – perhaps she longed for a child herself. But I just told it how it was for me. Danny was the bringer of joy, the encapsulation of all that was lovable and beautiful and tender. For the first time, I appreciated the profound secular meaning of the Christian nativity scene: to worship a baby in a cold, dark world is like suddenly finding new hope and light and love. The whole world is transformed.

Ingrid and I would meet up weekly, sometimes with the other antenatal group mothers and babies, and sometimes just together with Jack and Danny, asleep in their car seats or latched on for a feed. The babies smiled on cue at six weeks, gained weight and absorbed our hearts and minds so much that the world outside seemed to recede into the distance.

Yet midwinter was all around. Nothing grandiose or historic was happening in our comfortable corner of North London. There was food on the table, Nick was writing his second book, we were financially secure. And yet within weeks, the left side of Danny's face started twitching and he was showing muscle weakness down his neck, left shoulder and arm. I felt the cold nighttime of anxiety for Danny start to creep in when the doctor referred him to a paediatrician for these symptoms, which were a greater worry at that time than the fact that he seemed to find it so very hard to digest his milk.

During these months, my mother would phone and tell me of her concerns for my father and his increasing confusion – which turned out to be the onset of dementia. I was torn between the undertow of these dual anxieties and the desire to hold on to all the good around us. How to carry these worries with lightness, so as not to feed the dark, while at the same time giving them due attention? To be grateful for the comfort and the security we were lucky enough to experience, while at the same time meeting the challenges of the future head-on?

There was much to be grateful for. And in retrospect, what stands out at the top of the list of good luck – our family's, as well as that of Ingrid, Hugh and Jack – is this: we had brilliant GPs. Our homes happened to be within the catchment area of a truly outstanding doctor's practice that never, ever failed us. From the first new-birth visit to our home, and the regular baby clinics at the surgery, through to the more specific and costly demands we would all be making on the practice in due course, our families benefited from a truly excellent manifestation of the NHS at its best. All the doctors seemed kind and hard-working, as did the nurses, healthcare assistants and receptionists. I couldn't help noticing also that the senior partner, who combined academic and clinical work, was resolutely opposed to the idea of turning the NHS into a market.

Danny was assigned to Dr P. If we could have asked for the perfect GP, the answer would have been this dark-haired Irishman who listened attentively and with a stillness that made you think you were the only patient he had to see that day. And who, having listened, made you feel better just by the comforting, gentle tone of his voice.

In those early days I had no way of knowing the extent of this enormous piece of luck that had come our way. But even then there was gratitude, because we visited the surgery more regularly than your average mother and baby. And each time, I came out wanting to don the old badge from my student nursing days in the 1980s that said: 'I ♥ NHS.'

★

In the first two months of his life, Danny's facial asymmetry, the weakness of the muscles on his left side and the slight twitch of his face became temporarily overshadowed by an impending operation to repair hernias on both sides of his groin. He would have to undergo a general anaesthetic.

Danny's Auntie Gill (Nick's sister), on hearing that Danny's first return to hospital was thus to take place in December 1993, sent him a soft toy of Raymond Briggs's beloved Snowman as a companion. This act of giving precisely the right thing at the right time, of solidarity and compassion, was entirely characteristic of her. But even Gill could not have foreseen how big a role this and successor Snowmen would play in Danny's later life. For there have been more Snowmen since that first soft toy of December 1993, growing larger as Danny himself has grown. Nowadays they have to be custom-made and ordered in bulk so that as one wears out, another is ready to step in, to be his constant bedfellow, pillow, comforter and support. Three smaller ones perch on his living-room windowsill. During the first Covid-19 lockdown, when Danny was unable to see his family through week after interminable week, he took all of them to bed with him.

Just one sufficed at the time of his hernia repair.

My previous nursing experience made me determined to be matter-of-fact about the operation. After all, it was not complicated or life-threatening surgery. Because of this gung-ho attitude, Nick and I jointly agreed that it would be sensible if only one of us was with Danny during his brief stay in hospital. That way, Nick would be able to stay at home enjoying, for the first time in several weeks, an opportunity to write without the usual distractions of a young baby and wife in a small house, and I would handle the parallel work of being with Danny at Queen Elizabeth Hospital.

In my sleep-deprived daze and determined optimism, I had managed to forget that prior to surgery a patient has to be 'nil by mouth' for several hours, and I was totally unprepared for the impact of this starvation on a twelve-week-old baby who was used to breastfeeding on demand. After ten minutes of Danny's crying, it was heart-rending. Within thirty minutes it was torture. Hours later, it was hell. Inevitably, the wait was longer than planned, and it felt as if Danny's lungs would burst and both our hearts would break from his despair – at being held by a mother who refused to feed him. Sometimes other mothers would hold him for me, thanks to the solidarity that often dwells in the territory of distress.

Some may wonder, did this have a long-lasting impact on Danny, and, if so, what kind of impact? Did he learn, early in his precious life, that his mother was a monster, who on the one hand nurtures and feeds and cherishes him, and on the other – apparently wilfully – withholds all of this and lets him starve despite his desperate cries? I wonder, too, if those people who persist in believing that autism and learning disability may be the result of early emotional trauma will seize on those hours at Queen Elizabeth Hospital as cast-iron evidence of their theory with regard to Danny.

Back then we knew nothing of the future diagnosis that awaited us, or the medical problems that would accompany it in his case. But if I had been asking myself at that time what trauma I might have inflicted on him, Danny gave me full reassurance when the effects of the general anaesthetic wore off. It was as if the rigours of the previous starving hours, and the surgery itself, had never happened. He smiled, he gurgled, he didn't seem to mind that he was in a hospital cot rather than at home; he was our beautiful, cheerful, beaming baby, greeting each new waking hour with trust and pleasure. He would go on giving the answer as he grew up, revealing an ability to build strong attachments and a positive nature that would embrace the good times with contagious joy despite all the suffering that would accompany him on his journey.

★

Danny was the sweetest baby, and coped stoically with the medical investigations that took place during the first two years

of his life: the MRI scan that could find no explanation for the
left-sided facial twitch and the weakness of neck, shoulder and
arm that delayed his crawling; the hypermobile ankle joints.
Then came a sudden decline in verbal progress at the age of
seventeen months, the replacement of some early words with
guttural and repetitive sounds, and a persistent avoidance of
social engagement. Danny cried when new people came too
close, preferring to flick through picture books or play with his
shape sorter, over and over again as if nothing else in the world
could interest him.

Sometimes he seemed to zone out completely. Whereas Jack
would turn at the sound of a police car and say 'nee-naw
nee-naw', Danny wouldn't stir. It was as if he had not heard,
despite having passed a hearing test. At swimming sessions for
babies and toddlers, Jack would splash about, while Danny lay
still in my arms, apparently uninterested.

This list of issues conveys Danny-the-baby-with-problems,
Danny-the-bringer-of-worry. But through all of this, despite all
the worry, Danny was *wonderful*, and fully intact in the unique
person that he is.

He thrilled at physical interaction with Nick and me, as we
blew raspberries on his tummy, or jiggled him up and down.
Throughout infancy and toddlerhood he loved rough-and-
tumble, being swung and whirled around. He had a lovely sense
of humour and a heart-melting smile. Watching Nick while he
put CDs on the shelf or snipped at the vine covering our
kitchen lean-to would send Danny into fits of chuckles, then
giggles, then uncontrollable laughter as he delighted in whatever it was that was so hilarious about what Nick was doing.
When Danny woke in the mornings, the dawn chorus was his
cheerful chirruping and burbling – the best sound in the world.
Sometimes in the night we would suddenly hear peals of laughter, as if someone had told him a brilliant joke. We would say
fondly that he was talking to his angels. Along with 'mama' and

'diddle' (for 'mummy' and 'daddy'), one of his first words was
'duddle' – meaning 'cuddle', which in turn meant 'I want to be
lifted up for a cuddle.'[1]

From an early age Danny experienced joy when being swung.
We would sit him in baby-swings which we gently pushed, and
he gradually progressed to those with less protection, and then,
over the years, ultimately, to regular swings, which still to this
day elicit sounds of joy, whoops of delight and a smile of transported happiness. He shared his pleasure with others in the
early days. At a park where there were adjacent toddler-sized
swings, he would grin at his fellow swingers as they flew back
and forth beside him, as if to say, 'Isn't this just *the best thing*?'
Such attention to others and sharing of pleasure didn't chime
well, I later discovered, with textbook autism.[2]

But then a lot of autistic people's experiences belie the
textbooks.

2

AN INTRODUCTION TO AUTISM

Danny finally acquired the diagnosis of autism and global developmental delay just before his third birthday. The GP had gently urged a referral to the local community paediatrician, who in turn referred him for a multidisciplinary assessment.

I had already researched autism, in response to the concerns of local health professionals and the widening gap between Danny's development and that of his peers, so the diagnosis came as no surprise.

What did it mean, back then, to say that someone was autistic?

If you wanted to go down the official, technical route, you could refer to two contrasting sets of criteria by which autism was diagnosed. One was the World Health Organization's *International Statistical Classification of Diseases and Related Health Problems* (ICD), and the other was the American Psychiatric Association's *Diagnostic and Statistical Manual of Mental Disorders* (DSM). Both were updated at periodic intervals, and at the time I became 'autism aware', we were on ICD-10 and DSM-IV.[1] (The numbers 10 and IV reveal how many versions and updates preceded them.) Diagnosis could be conferred only by medical experts who had been trained to identify these criteria in the people presenting to them.

If you read books written by psychiatrists and psychologists, it is most likely you would be told that there was an undoubted genetic contributor to autism, which in turn influenced the development, structure and wiring of the brain. The impact on the brain would lead to observable characteristics that were collectively referred to as the 'triad of impairments'.[2] This triad consisted of deficiency in three key areas: communication, social interaction and imagination, and these three in turn underlay a frequently observed pattern of restricted and repetitive behaviours.

This was all very well, but it wasn't a catchy or memorable description, and it didn't make for easy understanding, let alone explanation, for most of us who were, of course, untrained in the esoteric world of diagnostic procedures and categories.

'My son has autism.'

'Oh, really? What actually is autism?'

'It means he has the triad of impairments.'

'Er, what?'

'Well … it means he has difficulties communicating, and with social interaction, and behaves in unusual ways.'

You can see how this might not have been enlightening to the casual enquirer. The problem was that it was so unspecific. You could reel off all the criteria and still know very little about the condition.

None of this was straightforward. It seemed that an array of unique and contrasting people could earn and share the diagnosis of autism, however different from one another they appeared to be. Some were happy to be around other people, some weren't; some developed good language skills, while others struggled even to use sign language; some displayed intense curiosity in their environment, while others (like Danny) seemed to zone out. In particular, for example, the triad's psychological/psychiatric origins seemed to downplay the highly *physical* role of self-stimulatory behaviour or 'stimming'. For many young children this meant repeated flapping of arms, twiddling of fingers or bigger movements such as sudden jumping or clasping of hands. For older autistics, and those with greater language and intellectual skills, there may still be a need to rock, or fiddle with an object, in a way that critics felt was meaningless and freaky, but which others held as necessarily soothing or expressive, and a great source of pleasure.[3]

And then there was the issue of intellectual ability. On the one hand you might meet someone with so-called low-functioning autism (LFA), generally characterised by learning disability, also known as 'intellectual disability'. These terms replaced 'mental retardation' as it used to be called in the UK and, until 2010, in the USA.[4] On the other hand, you might meet an autistic person with strong intellectual abilities, and this would earn them the description of high-functioning autism (HFA). And to add to the confusion, there was another condition called Asperger syndrome (AS), which was similar in some respects to, but at that time officially considered to be distinct from, HFA. At the point at which I became autism aware, academics and clinicians were debating whether this was a real or artificial distinction.

Difficulties in explaining or describing autism, unease and discomfort around what autism is, have intensified with each passing year. Not merely among those of us who are not employed in clinical or scientific fields, but also among the 'experts'. At the time of Danny's diagnosis, enquiry into what might be *a* (or *the*) key feature of autism was in full swing. Attempts to get to the crux of autism were expanding in fields such as genetics, neurology, neurobiology, neuroscience and molecular psychiatry. Several explanatory psychological/cognitive models were put forward, relating to theory of mind,[5] central coherence[6] and executive functioning.[7] Some of these were helpful when trying to understand the world from an autistic person's point of view, but there were many times when they fell short. All would later be questioned or qualified.[8] There would be multiple theories to explain what autism is and how it impacts on people, and even a questioning as to whether 'autism' is a valid category at all.[9] This is fascinating and bewildering in equal measure. There has been a proliferation of both scientific investigation and conceptual debate in the field throughout Danny's lifetime. I feel privileged to have been an observer and occasional participant in all of this.

In those days, when I turned to writing not by clinicians but by laypeople (parents, mostly), I was told that having an autistic child was incredibly hard work and that professionals would rarely understand or take our ideas seriously enough. Perhaps in time our children might learn to speak, to read, to be part of a wider community, albeit with many unusual differences in focus and behaviour, or perhaps they would find a way of communicating through signs or pictures. But whatever the outcome would be, these parent stories informed me that it would be a long, hard slog with little support.[10]

As far as I was aware, there were very few books by autistic adults, but I had heard of two, by Temple Grandin[11] and Donna Williams.[12] Both were far more gifted than the autism stereotype of learning-disabled, mute and destructive children – not only were they functioning adults but also they could write books, for heaven's sake! In addition, there was the film *Rain Man*,[13] which helped familiarise the public with the idea that an autistic person could be simultaneously disabled and gifted.

Danny didn't seem to have much in common with any of these people.

Despite the inability to get a simple explanation from the clinicians at the point of Danny's diagnosis, we were fortunate at least in that we weren't given the third degree. If the diagnosis had taken place in the 1960s, 1970s or early 1980s, the experience would have been nothing short of a nightmare. In those days, toxic ideas about the causes of autism held sway. So-called 'refrigerator mothers' (cold, perfectionist or harbouring subconscious hostility towards their babies) were blamed for their children's symptoms. Recommended treatment thus consisted of 'parentectomy' – removing the children from their parents. Bruno Bettelheim's popularisation of this fantasy dominated thinking for decades.[14]

Thankfully, some brave and clever parents fought back against the prevailing beliefs. In the USA, Bernard Rimland is credited with leading the way in this important struggle,[15] and in the UK, Michael Baron, Lorna Wing and colleagues set up what became the National Autistic Society (NAS). A psychiatrist by profession, Lorna Wing led research that highlighted the breadth of the autism spectrum. Subsequent advances in genetic and psychological science confirmed that autism was organic – rooted in biology rather than emotional trauma. And from then on, the research endeavour into the genetics and cognitive features of autism mushroomed almost exponentially.[16]

By the time it was our turn to go through the diagnostic process, Nick and I just had to sit through many appointments answering over and over again the same questions about Danny, his birth history, our family histories, his early development, while Danny got restless in the background or – more often – sat contented and self-contained, rhythmically turning the pages of his picture books.

3

No Man's Land

I have often been asked how I felt once the diagnosis arrived, in the summer of 1996.

Mixed, is the answer. I was profoundly conflicted.

On the one hand I remember crying with my two oldest school friends. I have since interrogated those tears. Why did I cry? Not because Danny had changed or was any the less loved. He was, if anything, even more loved. Perhaps I cried because I was mourning the end of one version of our imagined future. Perhaps I was sad because I believed that Danny would experience more struggle and distress over the course of his life than would most of his peers.

On the other hand, I was relieved to have a new sense of purpose. Now we could start figuring out how best to help Danny thrive in a world that was not a hospitable place for him. Even while Nick and I knew that Danny would be cherished by us for the rest of our lives, we sensed that his difference from the norm would mark him out in the eyes of many as socially deficient in some ways, as lesser, flawed, even not fully human. And I felt ready to tell the world that it was wrong to think like this.

Yet Danny's diagnosis was only one of the changes we were dealing with, and I think my tears were shed for all of the other changes too. All three members of our small family were on a journey that seemed to propel us into a new landscape at speed. Some of these changes were marvellous, but still they required resilience and adaptation. For example, Nick had gone from being a little-known writer to the author of two bestsellers and a weekly column in the *Independent on Sunday*. The film rights to *High Fidelity*, his first novel, had been sold, and he and his friends David Evans and Amanda Posey were immersed in transforming a fictionalised account of *Fever Pitch* into a film that would star Colin Firth. Yet Nick was also having to cope, behind this outward success, with deep anxiety about his adored Danny, and a wife who increasingly felt that her own life was spiralling.

My father's condition had deteriorated to the point where my mother, despite her best efforts, was not able to look after him safely. A hospitalisation in early 1996 signalled that he was never to come home. We found a nursing home where he would stay until his death in 1997. His was a long and poignant farewell. He had been well enough for long enough to forge a bond with little Danny, who saw something magnetically wonderful in this benevolent silver-haired man whose eyesight and mind were failing him. Memories of the two of them at the height of their connection – these two sweet-natured, gentle souls bound together both in bloodline and in qualities of character – are precious. But the special bond was bound to break, once the dementia took an ever stronger hold on my father, and as Danny sank deeper into his own regression.

I then left my job.

It made total sense that, in the event of Danny's childcare arrangements proving unsustainable, it would be me rather than Nick who would be the full-time parent. I was an eminently replaceable part-time researcher on a fledgling project about GP fundholding, earning not much, whereas Nick was … well, he was becoming a cultural force.

And Danny's childcare arrangements did prove to be unsustainable. Angeline, his nanny, was lovely. She looked after Danny with as much devotion as she did her own child – Iona, a little girl of a similar age. Danny's early speech (before the regression) included the word 'eeya', which meant 'here you are', copying what was clearly a frequent tendency of Iona and Angeline to give things to him and to include him in everything they did. Brilliant. Danny and Iona were driven around in a double buggy, to music groups and playgrounds. Friends who saw them out together commented on how harmonious it all seemed.

But in February 1995, Angeline and Iona abruptly returned to Scotland, and Danny seemed to retreat from the world. The possibility that their departure somehow inflicted irreparable soul-damage on Danny was a prominent worry for Nick and me. We eventually agreed that, given Danny's increasingly distressed-seeming behaviour, it would be wrong to require him to adapt to another change in his care.

I tendered my resignation and, to my great surprise, found myself weeping uncontrollably not just in front of my boss but also on my own in my office for the rest of the day. I felt that a tornado had lifted me, like Dorothy in *The Wizard of Oz*, up out of my previous life and dropped me into in a new land. In time I might be able to draw on sufficient resources of courage, heart and intellect, but right now – like the lion, tin man and scarecrow – I was too disoriented to believe this was possible. My professional identity was in pieces and, apparently, there was very little of me left.

Yet Danny was very much with us, and in the safety of our home he continued to enjoy the bouncing and swinging and music and cuddles that were the key features of our happy inter-action with him. Although he was seemingly content on his own for hours, flicking pages of books and doing his jigsaw puzzles, or rocking on the sofa as he watched over and over again his favour-ite videos (of Pingu, Fireman Sam, Postman Pat), he was unceas-ingly affectionate and relished rough-and-tumble, smiling and squealing with delight and enjoying frequent cuddles.

But, aside from the release offered by swings in public parks, this side of Danny was rarely on display outside the home. More often, when out, as Nick later described in a newspaper article,[1] he would be 'slumped on a parental shoulder', silent and expressionless. If we took him to see friends – even Ingrid and Jack – he would make his desire to be back home very clear, by standing by the front door. Despite many inducements (crisps, his favourite book, a bunch of keys or bouncing and swinging games), he would calmly but persistently return to his front-door vigil. Usually he was relatively patient. There were no tantrums or meltdowns, just this persistent and insistent declaration that he didn't want to be anywhere, or with anyone, other than with his mum and dad at home.

Later – decades later – I would read that the idea of 'normal' child development was a relatively recent phenomenon dating from the early twentieth century.[2] I would read a lot about how atypicality is not the same thing as inferiority, that difference need not mean you are substandard or in need of fixing. And I could have found hope at that time, if I had known where to look, in the early manifestations of what would become the neurodiversity movement. In North America, Jim Sinclair had launched Autism Network International in 1992, and in the Netherlands an email list called 'Independent Living on the Autism Spectrum', or 'InLv', was launched by a young autistic computer programmer called Martijn Dekker.[3] These were early signs of what in time would be a real community of autistics, and a movement that would transform the landscape. This might have shown me that, out there, attempts were being made to rehabilitate autism as a condition with strengths, not just difficulties, and to allow autistic people to frame their own priorities rather than be lamented by neurotypical (or 'NT') onlookers. But at the point at which Danny's diagnosis finally came, in the summer of 1996, autism was presented to us only in terms of deficits and absences. It was Bad News.

I would later read also about how painful it was for autistic people to imbibe from an early age the pessimism with which their condition was viewed. And certainly the discourse at the time reinforced the notion that having an autistic child was awful. The word 'tragic' featured in a letter written to my mother by one of her friends when she heard the news of Danny's diagnosis.

Likewise, the impact on parents was often conveyed in entirely negative terms, and certainly I recognised that my life had been blown off course. Normal outlets for mothers with young children were closed to me, because Danny doggedly avoided interactive play. I was isolated in a kind of no mother's land, different from my peers in both professional and maternal experience, and with few reference points or goals to guide me. If only I had known then what I know now: that what lay ahead was an opportunity and a privilege offered to few – to meet a whole new group of people, to learn and grow and find new purpose and interest. To appreciate to the full the freedom of not having to conform. And to continue to be besotted with Danny, to find pleasure and love and comfort in his presence, to want no other son but him, for the rest of my days.

4

KIDZMANIA

Other than park swings, there were few places outside the home where Danny could be guaranteed to enjoy himself. The exception was Kidzmania, a former warehouse converted into an indoor soft play centre whose cavernous interior was cladded with colourful and sturdy plastic cushioning. With its collection of rope ladders, mirrors and mazes it offered a paradise of discovery and adventure. Here, excited children crawled through tunnels and negotiated bridges, scaled climbing frames and raced down slides. They would call out to one another and shout, chasing, pushing, tumbling, while parents and childminders could sit, drink coffee and chat, letting their charges roam free.

Yet I would be on red alert. Danny never left my sight for a second. He was physically slower than the other children, gentler and more cautious, and although his smiles and exploration showed that he enjoyed himself, I knew he would not be able to negotiate any misunderstandings or collisions with the other children. Even in this safest of places, he might need my protection and intervention.

We would go there frequently, particularly on rainy days, when sodden park swings lost their attraction. I tried to avoid the busiest times, when the noise and hurly-burly would be too much for his senses. But even in these quieter slots, there was no avoiding other children. And because of this, Danny and I were given an early initiation into the world of disability – both the ways in which it can impact on the individual and also its ability to elicit widely contrasting responses from other people.

Incident 1

Danny had ventured slowly up a ladder to the top of a slide, then stopped, and sat. And sat. And sat. He had a serene smile on his face, and he waved his arms in his familiar animated stim. Behind him, the queue of waiting children grew longer, and I could see the puzzled looks on some of their faces when he failed to move. I wondered how long it would take for their bewilderment to turn into impatience and then possibly into anger, while he deprived them of their chance to use the slide. Nothing for it but to push my way, as gently as possible, through to the ladder, then squeeze past each child as I climbed up to where Danny was sitting impervious to the queue at his back. As I arrived I heard the little boy behind Danny saying kindly: 'I said, "What's your name?"'

This was so sweet! It was apparent that this child had tried to engage Danny in conversation for quite a while now, hoping to find a way of connecting that might persuade Danny to launch himself down the slide, or establish the reason for this long wait and then jointly problem-solve. And Danny of course had not replied, nor even seemed to register this boy's existence, let alone his friendliness.

I calculated the relative pros and cons of coaxing Danny back down the ladder (but the long line of waiting children meant there was not enough room to manoeuvre) or softly pushing him down the slide. I chose the latter, and then followed him down. We both emerged unscathed.

Incident 2

In an enclosed area that led to more ladders and tunnels, Danny was momentarily alone. Another little boy entered the space, checked Danny out, homed in on his difference and vulnerability, and then, when he thought no one was looking, kicked him twice.

I rushed over to Danny and removed him from the situation. The perpetrator had by then escaped.

Incident 3

Here is Danny, sitting in the middle of the ball pond on his own, and until now he has been happy. Suddenly, and with no discernible cause, he starts to weep. I observed no trigger for this sudden distress, but it is palpable. My darling child is sitting alone and crying because of – as it seems to me – sudden over-whelm. It is as if he is saying, 'I am alone and I don't understand this place. I have tried so hard but I have exhausted my reserves of curiosity and adaptability. This is all too much.'

I swept him up and the distress abated as we drove home. But it left a lasting impression. God knows I have seen and heard Danny cry many times since. But there was something about his lonely weeping back then – such a small, innocent boy in the middle of a place that was supposed to be fun, in the middle of a world that had become alien to him – that broke my heart, as if I were glimpsing what might lie ahead.

The memory of these incidents has intensified over the years. I revisit them in technicolour, sound system pounding, emotions whirling around all over again. They have become almost alle-gorical, as reference points to guide my beliefs and actions, both as a mother who longs to protect her son and as an engaged citizen. They shed light on the ways in which other people can make such a difference to the disabled person, for good and bad.

Maybe no amount of social change can make everything better. But it is no exaggeration to suggest that the external conditions surrounding the disabled person can and do affect *almost* everything.[1] It is imperative to deal with the abuse that comes along, be this from individuals or institutions. Yet it is also imperative to be driven by the knowledge that adaptations – the 'reasonable adjustments' of equality law[2] – are not a utopian dream. They occupy the realm of the practical and the possible. There is a kind of defeatism in believing that the lone kicker sums up all that is probable. It is not naive to keep believing in the kindness of strangers.

5

On the Margins

In those early years I was often acutely aware of the difference between my experience of motherhood and that of others. Well-meaning people did not know what to say to me. Trying to be kind, they might tell me how marvellous I was in my handling of Danny. What I wanted to say back to them was, 'Look how marvellous *Danny* is. Why don't you try to find out more about *him*?' If they sympathised with my struggle, it felt like an insult to him. If they tried to reach out in some kind of solidarity, it all too often felt patronising or crass. It wasn't their intention, of course. It can be hard to find the right words.

At the same time, I was not unaware of the fact that being the mum of a child with Danny's unique qualities offered several advantages. For one, I did not have to worry about hosting children's birthday parties. This was something I had dreaded even when pregnant, being devoid of the requisite creative talent to magic up spell-binding entertainment, or to bake character-driven birthday cakes. Danny was content to have a small cake and a handful of cousins, to hear us sing 'Happy Birthday' and then escape. That's my boy! Many years later, whenever Ingrid phoned me on a Saturday morning, freezing on the edges of a godforsaken football pitch where little boys inexplicably enjoyed themselves in muddy competitive mayhem, I thanked Danny for his indifference to any kind of team sport. And projecting to the future, I could already acknowledge that Danny and I were sheltered from the usual pressures that go along with typical development – jostling for status, exam results, drugs, being called up in the event of war ...

And although Danny's and hence my sleep were permanently disrupted, we didn't experience the full repertoire of challenges that can be a feature of some autistic children's behaviour – children who, from a young age, are on a mission to run away, climb, bash things up, generally wreak havoc. A friend frequently had to call out the police and fire service, due to her autistic twins' various experiments with the kitchen cooker, the rooftops of neighbouring houses and nocturnal excursions to the local park. She nicknamed them, with a mixture of adoration, pride and exhaustion, Trouble and Mayhem. And heaven knows it's inconvenient when you've had to unblock the loo or call out the plumber/builder/locksmith for the umpteenth time, and it's horrid when your other children are weeping because once again their toys have been broken by their unruly sibling. And most of all it's heartbreaking when your autistic child is crying and screaming and wailing in some kind of existential-seeming despair for reasons you can't fathom, when they're hitting their head or biting their own arm, and when they push you away when all you want to do is to pick them up, hold them close and console them.

For families whose experience reflects this level of challenge, any positive assertion about autism and learning disability can be aggravating in the extreme. But nonetheless, the negative image is by no means true of all – or even most. And certainly Danny did not display the behaviours that cause parents such distress. He was chiefly interested in tapping things with the back of his hand (tabletops, windows, CD covers) and requisitioning objects that fascinated him. Keys had (and still have) particular allure, but so – in homes such as my mother's, where ornaments and trinkets were on display – did the tops of dainty teapot lids, shiny photo frames, collections of small shells. Many of these would turn up several days later in unexpected locations where he'd dropped them, suddenly bored or beguiled by the next compelling object.

Nick and I would relay with amused pride the more engaging departures from convention that Danny enjoyed: lying on top of a semi-naked sunbather in the park, or smiling broadly as he removed a pair of spectacles from the nose of an elderly lady in the doctor's waiting room. In time I would meet other parents with similar tales, usually recounted not as complaint but as sources of amusement – the secret club to which we belonged was full of humour and affection, alongside the other kaleidoscope of emotions. None of these things, as Charlotte Moore emphasises,[1] are tragic. They are inconvenient and sometimes embarrassing, but many worse things happen in the world.

The biggest challenge for all of us parents, however, is fear for the future. What will happen when the cuteness of childhood makes way for the ungainliness of adolescence? Unusual sounds from a toddler or child are quirky and endearing, but from a man with a deep voice they can be unsettling or even threatening. Meltdowns in a four-year-old are more easily explained than equivalently violent manifestations in a fully grown adult.

Parental fear grows with the discovery that not only are there individual bullies to contend with – the child who kicked Danny in Kidzmania – but also there can be institutional opposition writ large. One hears of abuses in adult care settings, and even deaths brought about by neglect or lack of training. The data is there, not to mention the horror stories that hit the headlines.[2]

We learn that despite an advanced economy, social care provision often falls well short of offering sufficiently skilled and well-resourced assistance, that schools can be inhospitable and punitive, that the wider community still doesn't know or think enough about how people who seem different can still be respected and loved and admired, possess strengths and abilities to contribute for all our benefit, have wonderful lives and teach us and enrich us, and that *we are all in this together*. Instead, parents are too often left to battle it out alone, sometimes demonising the very children they love most, even though in reality they are joint victims of external conditions that make them feel invisible and abandoned.

My point is this: fear for the future is caused chiefly by the societal inadequacies of the wider world, not by the child and their condition. In saying this, I am not trying to minimise the difficulties that accompany specific individual natures and impairments. Yet what I have learnt is that we need to broaden our focus, to recognise the significance of the wider social, economic, political landscape in shaping how we experience and respond to disability, and to think again about many things one might hitherto have taken for granted.

Even wealthy people, powerful in every other area of their lives, come up against situations and institutions that make them feel powerless, that turn them into supplicants at the limits of their own resources. They will have to persuade various arms of government, both local and central, that their child needs things 'the system' is not always willing to give. This may be the first time that middle- and upper-class people have ever had to come up against the welfare state and fight for entitlements. They are suddenly on the fringes, partly estranged from peers whose children are 'normal', and at least in part they are now shoulder to shoulder with other people who have to apply for benefits, maybe just to keep a roof over their heads, or to maintain an income hovering around the poverty line.

This newfound awareness is not altogether a bad thing! Despair when you hear that your child will no longer get speech therapy because of chronic skill shortages, or that your application for a new blue badge has been rejected even though your child's condition remains the same – these aggravations generate solidarity based on raw experience that extends beyond mere sympathy or imagination.

In addition to joining the ranks of people who apply for benefits, you appreciate firsthand the overwhelming necessity of high public spending on skilled professionals who work in education, health and social care. It is probable, even if you are a high-income earner, that your disabled child will cost the state far more than you contribute.

And then there are the underlying attitudes that you have to learn to address.

I think of several people I know who are struggling – often as they grow older – to get around, or to see or hear clearly. Yet they are determined to keep their use of glasses, or a hearing aid, to an absolute minimum. Somehow such aids signify weakness, fragility, something to be ashamed of, and this in turn undermines their self-respect. This is one small example of 'ableism', whereby disability is felt, almost reflexively, to be humiliating, lesser, eliciting diminished respect. Similarly, I have known people to recoil from the possible use of a wheelchair. 'I would feel really humiliated if I were in a wheelchair,' a friend once said, having broken her leg. Would she have felt comfortable articulating such a notion of humiliation in connection with other forms of human difference – for example, race, sex, sexual orientation or gender? But unconscious ableism can often slip in, even among the most progressive.

Disabled people are not conventional. Rather, they are, if anything, seen as an afterthought, to be pitied perhaps, or reviled. Worse, they are often not seen as fully human. Hate crimes against disabled people are rarely given media prominence, but they happen daily.[3]

Pity and despair are not the answers. Indignation about how badly the system can treat people includes a desire to reclaim a positive story. I want to shout from the rooftops that Danny is the best thing that has happened to me, and that having a disabled child can be truly wonderful, particularly if one is buoyed up by encouragement, assistance and helpful interest – the spirit the little boy in Kidzmania showed while he waited all those years ago, when Danny sat at the top of the slide. Even while part of our story will expose system failures, obstructions and abuses, these do not sum up the entire state of affairs. We don't hear enough positive or encouraging stories, about the autistic and learning-disabled people who go on to have happy, worthwhile lives. Their flourishing, not their oppression, is something about which the mainstream is often sadly unaware.[4]

This confidence in positive outcomes stems from a position of privilege. I am not fool enough to think I would be so certain had we not been supported financially, and had we not found permanent reason to trust that good people come along when you need them. Along with Danny's diagnosis and the challenges that lay ahead came a band of angels who would stay the course through decades. Like Sarah.

6

SARAH, AND THE CHALLENGE
OF INCLUSION

Sarah came into our lives when Danny was four months old. Our usual childcare arrangement had fallen through. I had only just returned to work, and I was unable to reschedule an important meeting with my three bosses. We called a relief nanny agency.

I needed to leave for work before anyone had arrived, thus leaving Nick in charge.

Once at the office, I immediately called him.

'How's it going?' I asked, fearing the worst.

'It's fine.'

This level of cheerful positivity was not what I'd expected.

'Really?'

'Yes, honestly.'

Sarah was then just nineteen years old, a registered nanny from New Zealand. I knew she must be brilliant if Nick sounded so swiftly confident in her.

In due course, she would lodge with Ingrid, Jack and Jack's new little brother Ben. Years later, she would provide early child care for Danny's younger half-brothers, not to mention ongoing guidance, meals, transport, companionship, advice and friendship for the whole extended family, as well as going on to run Danny's Facebook page.

Her ability to perform magic is summed up in the following story.

By the time Danny and Jack were seven or eight, Ingrid and Hugh – like Nick and me – had separated. Ingrid was determined to ensure that, regardless, Jack had a good time on his birthday. She organised a bowling party at our local alley, and made one of her famous chocolate cakes. I was to take some of the food and drink to the bowling alley in my car, with Danny sitting in the back in his usual seat. But disaster struck. Ingrid dropped the cake, and to give her time to repair it, she asked me to take three little girls in my car instead. One little girl joined me in the front, and the other two shared the back seat with Danny.

I should have moved Danny to the front seat. I knew he hated the sound of children's high-pitched voices, that he found their animated conversation particularly hard on the senses, and that things that moved unexpectedly were a cause of alarm. He had never had anyone under the age of twenty sit beside him in the back seat, let alone two excited and talkative little girls.

But in the moment, my powers of anticipation failed me and the inevitable happened. About thirty seconds into the drive, Danny pinched the little girl sitting next to him. Pinched hard, and pinched again.

After the indignant exclamation of 'He pinched me!' a heavy silence fell upon us all. I could sense the girls' outrage and their shared dislike of this nasty boy who was bigger than them and who should know better. I also knew that if I reproached Danny in any way, it would cause him further distress and there was serious danger of a full-on meltdown, during which he would likely pinch again, or do something worse. They must have thought I was an even greater monster than Danny for not doing anything, other than to mutter, 'I'm so sorry, I don't think he meant to hurt you.' If I were to stop the car (where, on a red route?) to instigate a change of seating plan, this too might exacerbate his behaviour. So silence offered the best bet for reaching our destination safely.

Sarah was there to greet a troubled Danny and three furious little girls, while I went and found somewhere to park and sob.

I have no idea what Sarah said or how she pulled it off, but by the time I joined them in our bowling lane minutes later, the girls were cheering Danny as he pushed the ball down the ramp, insisting he should be given extra turns, and generally treating him like a king, with Sarah calmly and benignly in control.

I learned some important lessons about inclusion that day. In the car I had been thinking, 'It's all very well, this inclusion thing, but it just can't work. It ends in tears. For everyone.' But by the time the girls were thrilling at Danny's success (of which he seemed oblivious), I thought: 'Wow, this is fabulous. The girls are getting even more out of this than Danny is.'

Later it struck me how crucial Sarah's intervention had been in turning the situation around, and what this says about how inclusion can work well – *if* the person facilitating and guiding it is as skilled as Sarah. You need to have enough Sarahs to make it work, people with the right knowledge, experience and attitude. And this is only likely to come about, of course, if the Sarahs are given professional status and decent pay.

When Jack's bowling party was over, there was just enough time to take Danny to his usual Saturday late-afternoon venue: our local authority swimming pool. Here we could join the weekly session specifically and exclusively set aside for disabled people and their families and carers. I remember the wave of relief that came over me, now I was amongst my own tribe. After the stresses of a 'mainstream' children's party, I could now sit here with Danny and others in the jacuzzi, happy to survey the diverse ways in which the swimmers expressed their enjoyment – without inhibition, safe from the fear of being judged or ridiculed. Despite what I had learned about the possibility of positive inclusion, I couldn't fail to notice the greater comfort I felt in this segregated place.

And here I offer you one of the ways in which the world cannot be summed up in polarised positions of belief or allegiance. I have described how lonely I felt in the mainstream, with my very unusual son. I have acknowledged how soothing it was to be with others who were similarly different. And yet, I reject the idea that Danny and I, and those like us, should be consigned to the margins, forever sidelined as an invisible minority.

In cleaving to both things, am I guilty of doublethink? Do I want Danny and me to have our cake and eat it? Or, rather, am I simply highlighting the fact that meeting human needs is a complex and evolving endeavour, one that doesn't adhere to a static idea of the good life? That all of us – disabled and able, neurodivergent and neurotypical – require a range of approaches in order to thrive. We need to be challenged and stimulated, but we also need sanctuary. It can be both/and, rather than either/or. And then there's the question of 'rights'. Danny had every right to be part of Jack's party – to have deliberately not invited him would have been unthinkable. And thanks to Sarah, reasonable adjustments were duly made so that it all ended well. But he also had a right to attend a segregated swimming session. Why subject him to the crowded, noisy hurly-burly of an open session, which would be like some kind of torture for him, when he could enjoy the peace and freedom of our gentle disabled time?

Part 2

CONNECTIONS AND CAMPAIGNS

'The problem with pounding a square peg
into a round hole is not that the hammering
is hard work. It's that you're destroying the peg.'

Paul Collins, *Not Even Wrong: A Father's
Journey into the Lost History of Autism*

For some parents, the quest for interventions to help their autistic children takes on a campaigning fervour. Sometimes the focus of this fervour remains the child, and the child alone. At other times, it expands into a wider arena, where the struggle for one individual develops into a struggle for many. Common ground and shared experiences and beliefs – about what causes autism, or what intervention might help – generate solidarity. New groups are formed and parents can often drift into new friendships and allegiances that separate them from former acquaintances.

In trying to help Danny, I found myself propelled into a new campaigning role, in which a lot of my energy was devoted to trying to bring about what I believed to be positive change. In this way, being the mother of Danny required me to assume a persona I still don't fully recognise – a persona that can draw on the advantage of 'good connections' and move in influential circles, while never forgetting the role of chance and luck, and how ephemeral these privileges might turn out to be.

7

EARLY INTERVENTION

In 1996, when Danny was three and newly diagnosed, we started to be inundated with suggestions as to how to 'intervene'. By this I mean we were sent articles about different amazing potions, diets, therapies, philosophies, you name it, that would help Danny overcome his difficulties. Some said they would lead him to 'recover' from his autism.

The only thing about which the sensible-seeming experts agreed was the importance of autism-specific education. For some, if they were intellectually able enough, a mainstream school might meet a child's needs, as long as the teachers adjusted their approach and understood enough about autism. (Not many did, at that time.) For someone like Danny, with his learning disability already apparent, the experts advised a specialist environment: a structured timetable, high teacher–pupil ratios and teachers who knew about autism and could tailor their approach to the specific needs of each unique pupil.

And here is where we hit our first brick wall. Everyone was telling us that this was what Danny needed. And yet such provision was very hard to find. There was – and still is – massive under-provision.[1] We were, in relative terms, lucky. There was a local autism school, and there were local special schools. Danny would not be required, as so many other children were, to be bussed out of his local community to a school an hour or more away, or alternatively placed in a local school that was autism oblivious, where he might be kept safe (on a good day) but learn nothing, and, moreover, possibly feel overwhelmed, distressed, frightened.

But – the big but: although Danny was lucky enough to access a full-time place in an excellent nursery attached to the local special school, he made no discernible progress. The head teacher allowed me to go with him for the first fortnight, then gently suggested that it would be best if I faded out. This was fine, but on and off I would go back to observe, and I noticed that several of the other pupils had made visible strides, acquiring greater communication and social ability, evidently happy and thriving. Danny, on the other hand, was impenetrable. He rarely seemed to be upset, but it was as if he had shut down. No happy sounds, no sad sounds, no range of facial expressions and not even a stim as far as I can remember. Just blankness.

Meanwhile, the full-time nature of the nursery place gave me time to research, to read the articles people sent me, talk to those who knew others whose children had done amazingly well thanks to therapy X and intervention Y. I was part sceptical, part gullible. The list of things I dipped into includes cranio-sacral therapy (pleasant), holding therapy (don't get me started on that particular horror story[2]), Auditory Integration Therapy (baffling and with no apparent benefit for Danny), Hanen (seemingly ineffectual for Danny) and Lacanian psychotherapy (just one ghastly session was more than enough).

I have no quarrel with cranio-sacral therapy. Danny would relax while a therapist gently massaged his head. Danny loves massage to this day, and sometimes directs other people's hands to his head for deep pressure. What it did not do, despite some of the hype, was re-calibrate his neurology in any discernible way. Holding therapy, on the other hand, was a nightmare, based on the discredited theory that autism was an attachment disorder, and that forcing a child to bond by holding him and requiring eye contact would somehow cancel out his autism. After two sessions in which Danny wanted to break free from this way of being held, I came to my senses and realised that my bond with Danny was just fine in any case, and that he freely sought and responded to cuddles without recourse to planned, forced, 'bonding' sessions.

Auditory Integration Therapy required Danny to look at a screen in a small darkened room while listening to sounds on headphones. Some parental testimonials were enthusiastic. I remain sceptical, not just because Danny seemed uninterested, but because I imagine that the children who enjoyed the sessions might well have been able to appreciate similar sensory experiences more cheaply at home, without the intervention of 'therapists' and 'special equipment'. In Danny's case, I would say he tolerated rather than enjoyed the sessions.

The Hanen programme is favoured by many in the speech therapy profession and Danny, Nick and I duly attended four group sessions in our local health centre. We received positive feedback from the speech therapist based on our filmed interaction with Danny. We were apparently 'doing everything right', yet saw no change in his ability to communicate, or motivation to interact, even over several months. This was dispiriting, but not as crushing as the Lacanian episode, at the end of which I was informed that Danny was neither autistic nor experiencing developmental delay. Rather, I was told, any developmental problems in the family were those of his parents.

Years later, I would have been able to go to the Research Autism website,[3] where one could find hundreds of interventions for autism, some of which had encouraging evidence, some of which had none, and some of which were graded as actively harmful. That website did not exist when Danny was a child. But finally I stumbled across something that the website would rate relatively positively. This something was an approach entitled, unhelpfully, 'EIBI' or Early Intensive Behavioural Intervention. Within autism circles, it is most often referred to (not entirely accurately) under an umbrella term, 'ABA', which in turn stands for Applied Behaviour Analysis. I didn't know immediately, but these initials would dominate our lives for the next two decades.

ABA weaves its way in and out of our story like a snake, with – as the ancient myths and symbols imply – the dual potential for life and transformation, and for poison and harm.

When I embarked on a quest to find out more about ABA, I had no idea what I was letting myself in for.

8

ABA: Good News?

At this point I ask the reader to bear with me. Danny's and my story is not just about ABA and it most certainly will not lead inexorably to a conclusion that is unequivocally favourable to ABA. Nor, though, is it going to be a hatchet job.

I need to say this right away, because much of the discussion 'out there' requires one to take sides and to pursue a *pro* or *anti* standpoint with missionary zeal. If you look up ABA on the internet, you may well find that it is described *either* as the best – or indeed only – way to support an autistic child to become all they can be, *or* as a pernicious attempt to crush an autistic child's spirit and effect a traumatic reprogramming towards 'normality'.

Is there room for both to be true, or do they both misrepresent a far more complex picture? Can reality embrace both possibilities at once? And do I have to take sides on the battlefield that ABA has become?

Let me mark out the terrain, so that you can appreciate the contours of the landscape ahead.

★

When I started to explore interventions for Danny, all I knew
was what I had read, and what I had heard. What I had read was
this: in the USA, ABA was establishing itself as an intervention
for which medical insurance companies were willing to pay.
This was based chiefly on the practice and research conducted
by Ivar Lovaas and colleagues, relating to a pre-school
programme for autistic children conducted in the child's home.[1]
A follow-up study years later suggested that – as a result of this
approach to teaching and learning – nearly half the group
managed to access mainstream school and appear 'indistinguishable from their peers'.[2] This contrasted dramatically with a
comparison group who had not received the intervention.

I had also heard that behavioural intervention was often
dehumanising – using methods not dissimilar to dog training,
based on rewards for behaviour desired by the adult, and punishment for behaviour that the adult wanted to discourage.

Yet ABA kept entering into conversations. Three times it was
recommended to me, and three times I ignored the recommendations. Finally, I decided to see for myself what ABA had to
offer.

★

I am visiting a family to witness an ABA programme. All my
prejudices, all the rumours about this approach, are being overturned by the spectacle in front of me.

This lovely little autistic child is bursting with enthusiasm
and delight, bouncing up and down with eager excitement, as
he and his tutor work through round after round of learning
activities. He whoops with pleasure after naming correctly a
series of pictures held up on a board in front of him. He smiles
and cheers alongside his tutor when he responds correctly to
instructions, each delivered in short, consistent phrases. He has
learned the meaning, and the articulation, of over a hundred

words in the past few weeks. And he has lots of time to play, chill, spin or stim between each unit of work. He is having a total ball.

I have run out of reasons not to offer this approach to Danny.

★

Setting up home-based ABA programmes in the UK was hard. In contrast to parts of the USA and Scandinavia, where some areas had established centres of practice that employed consultants and tutors, the UK had few indigenous practitioners. Parents had to recruit tutors and find a consultant and/or supervisor to train them from scratch, and this usually meant paying for experts from abroad. They also had to have enough space in their home, and be able to fund the programme themselves or approach the local authority to fund it. This latter task usually sent them into a nightmarish and conflict-ridden process, as if the first tasks weren't headache enough.

Yet Danny's ABA programme virtually fell into our laps. Nick and I were introduced to a delightful and resourceful woman called Vivien, who introduced us to Danny's first two tutors, Sid and Geoff. They rapidly built a strong rapport with Danny. They could see how much he enjoyed the physical sensation of twirling and spinning, so with impressive resources of stamina and enthusiasm, they offered their own equivalent of a fairground ride within the safe confines of our front room. Also, because Nick was by now earning well from his writing, I didn't even have to worry about how to fund the programme, so we started right away, in May 1997, very close to my thirty-ninth birthday.

How lucky were we!

Danny took to the new routine immediately. Each day when the bell rang, he would stand at the top of the stairs, waiting to see who it would be. I remember him peering round the banisters with an expectant smile, and then making his way down and cheerfully following them into the sitting room (turned education room).

What followed were sounds of sheer joy. From Danny there were constant giggles turning into shrieks of laughter and pleasure, whoops of enthusiasm and his favourite 'oy oy oy' expression. From the tutors came the continual thrill of praise and encouragement:

'Well done, Danny.'

'Danny, what a superstar.'

'You did it!'

What I heard from the sitting room, and frequently went in to observe directly, was remarkable. I saw relationships build: the interaction of an adult with a child, a child whose autism and severe learning difficulties were accepted, but whose potential to learn and enjoy life were believed in and nurtured. In Danny's smiles and sounds, and some rudimentary early words, I beheld the shining, luminous, soaring happiness of a three-year-old who at long last was finding learning fun, and *discovering that adults in addition to his parents could be rewarding and trusted*. At his nursery he was stoical but solemn and unreachable, yet in the sessions of learning opportunities that the ABA home programme offered, it was as if a light came on.

I have sometimes wondered if Danny's enjoyment was chiefly due to the sensory extravaganza offered by his trusted tutors, rather than to the structured learning plan and technical niceties of ABA. I ask myself this because I have heard so much negative talk about ABA – something that will emerge later in our story. But telling it how it truly was: Danny responded well to the process of breaking learning down into small repeated steps, a feature of his ABA programme. The positive experiences – the 'reinforcers' based on the things he enjoyed, such as a swing, a bounce, a sparkly toy, a crisp or verbal praise – came frequently with each small step. In this way, all the teaching was designed to make him feel successful, and to move with the flow of his preferences and in response to his behaviour. He was eager for interaction with his tutors and at ease with the steady, consistent way in which they helped him build new areas of comprehension and skill.

At first the reinforcers for his achievements were all tutor-led. Soon, though, he was able to choose from a range of reinforcers offered to him. And it also quickly became clear that some rewards for his learning were becoming intrinsic: he no longer relied on the reinforcement given to him by his tutors, but found an activity natural or pleasing in its own right. For example, he learned to appreciate jigsaw puzzles this way – starting with praise for fitting two pieces together, then needing praise only for bigger puzzles with more pieces, and finally focusing on and completing them independently with a triumphant smile. To this day, he becomes absorbed in larger puzzles, for long periods. And always there is his look of pleasure and pride on completion. When we do them together, he outpaces me.

Soon we took Danny out of the nursery he had been attending, so that he could have ABA tutors visit throughout the week. Instead of spending hour after hour at home watching one snippet of a video over and over again, or being persuaded against his will to go out, or being required to spend large amounts of time with other children who rarely understood him and in whom he had no interest – instead of all that, he was being stimulated, rewarded, offered a range of activities and new ways to learn. He was being prompted and encouraged to understand things that he'd not understood before, and he was becoming his cheeriest, most engaged self.

9

ABA: THE CONTROVERSY

The science of behaviour analysis was established and used to guide a whole range of social interventions, long before it became associated with a specific application with regard to autistic children. It is rooted in a reaction against Freudian dominance of the psychology profession, which (detractors argued) seemed to be reliant on a fictional or speculative model of how humans operate. The challengers, in response, sought to achieve empirical objectivity, by observing and measuring how living things behave. By the time I had come to learn about behaviour analysis, this original debate had been overtaken by a much more specific area of controversy with regard to autism.

There are several elements to the controversy, and I hope I will be forgiven for breaches of technical precision when I set out what I believe to be the core propositions of behaviour analysis.

First of all, if you look at the natural world, you can see that behaviour is everywhere – plants, insects, trees, animals, people. In the case of plants and trees, we can say with near certainty that behaviour is not conscious, but still, it happens. When plants turn to the sun, respond to nutrients in the soil, photosynthesise, these could all be conceptualised as 'behaviour'. In the case of higher-level animals and humans, we believe that our behaviour is subject to conscious control; we make choices, we learn to control (some) impulses. Just how much of our behaviour is truly conscious is a big debate in philosophy, neurology, psychology, tying in with questions about whether or not we have free will.

But regardless of this debate, few would dispute the fact that a lot of our learning and influencing is not brought about by the deliberate attempt of one person to manipulate another, and not always consciously chosen; it just happens, as an organic part of our interactions with our environment and influenced by the consequences associated with, or brought about by, our behaviour.

It is also apparent that this natural process can be harnessed and deliberately utilised for benign reasons: teaching, medicine, therapy are all professions that seek to impact on human behaviour in a positive way. Most professionals who use behavioural analysis as a basis for their practice are sincere in their belief that they are trying to help people and society, by targeting criminality or encouraging literacy, or by helping individuals reduce anxiety, tackle addiction, wear seatbelts. And to this end, the field of behaviour analysis has acquired a raft of strategies and techniques, a specialist vocabulary and a strong body of scientific research, to provide environments that support, and offer consequences that will encourage, behaviour that is desirable. The terminology often used here is that it is 'socially significant'.

But desirable to whom? Significant in what way? Because of course we can all feel uneasy about cynical attempts to condition behaviour – manipulative advertising, for example, or political brainwashing. And this contributes to the aversion towards behaviour analysis that many have held.

The second point of controversy is an empirical one. Do these principles really sum up how humans grow and develop and learn? Are other things at work that render a behavioural approach too simplistic? At one level, it is hard to reject the empirical claim entirely, because ample experiments in psychology have demonstrated the power of conditioning, and most of us can think of everyday examples (salivation at the smell of preferred foods, for example). The controversy heats up around how we perceive 'internal' or 'interior' behaviours, such as thoughts and feelings, or even biological stimuli such as hormonal changes. Can we be taught to behave 'on the outside' in one way, while inward behaviours such as thinking and feeling are completely different? If ABA can bring about a change in outward behaviour, might this be skin-deep only, and short term at best? Or might it achieve profound alterations of identity and self-perception?

This question is key when we start to understand ABA's impact with regard to autism. It's one thing to use ABA to help a drug addict come off heroin, or to help someone overcome a fear of flying so that they can go and see their relatives abroad, or to promote literacy among the learning disabled. It's quite another thing to deprive a person of access to what is important to them (stimming, for example), just because they differ from other people in a way that the practitioners (and wider society, you could say) don't like. And for sure, ABA's early delivery, particularly via the Lovaas approach, seemed to be geared to trying to stop children behaving in an autistic way, such that an optimal outcome was equated with making autistic children 'indistinguishable from their peers', which constituted 'recovery' from autism.

An even bigger concern than this was the way behaviour analysis was being practised. Electric shocks were initially used by Lovaas, until this kind of punishment was replaced with sharp 'no's. (An extreme case is the Judge Rotenberg Center in America, which has earned pariah status because of its continued use of highly aversive techniques.[1]) The possibility that such punitive measures merely push certain issues 'underground', causing trauma and despair, low self-esteem and a sense of powerlessness seemed not to be taken seriously, and/or it was felt that the goal of 'recovery' justified the means used.

As I have said, the field of ABA stretches way beyond autism, and actually even within autism it is used in many different ways.[2] But still, the term 'ABA' has for many critics become synonymous with a particularly rigid approach, and one which by the late 1990s had become the default early intervention model in much of the USA.

All these arguments would come to the fore as Danny grew up, and as my world opened up. But early on in our foray into ABA, they were distant concerns. What was there, right in front of my eyes, was Danny having a great time. The structured, deliberate, repetitive way of delivering the building blocks of his learning – copying, matching, sorting – were things he had not been able to learn spontaneously, but were now making sense. And in listening to his laughs and squeals of delight, I was *not* hearing the sound of Danny losing his autism – he was not working his way to some kind of 'recovery'. I was *not* hearing his tutors attempting to eliminate all of autism's revealing behavioural signs – rocking, arm waving, focusing with fascination on small shiny objects. And seeking a 'recovery' from autism was never, ever, my aim. The bad things I would read and hear about ABA did not apply in Danny's case.

And so, for a while, I became an unequivocal advocate. I threw myself into parental forums in which I would hear of children for whom the more traditional interventions on offer – largely speech therapy (if available) and an educational framework called TEACCH[3] – had proved ineffectual. In addition, the approach had higher expectations for what the child could achieve, something that was particularly helpful for those autistic children who had previously been written off as unteachable. For these children, like Danny, it was ABA to which they responded enthusiastically, and after which demonstrable progress was observed. Many learned to use words, to read and write, and their social interaction with others became more fluent. The frequency of distressed behaviours reportedly reduced. And when difficulties were encountered – for example, if learning plateaued or a particular area proved especially problematic – there seemed to be a vast repertoire of new ways to tackle the situation, backed up by published research.

However, what we enthusiastic pro-ABA parents did not recognise at the time was that many autistic children might have the potential to learn spontaneously; they may find independent learning inherently reinforcing, and hugely preferable to a relentless bombardment of stimuli and consequences coming at them from their tutors (something that characterised the Lovaas approach). Many autistic children could and would acquire literacy, numeracy, functional communication and so on without the apparatus of structured programmes and externally generated reinforcement. But parents like me tended to hear only of the children with learning disability, or those for whom a brief spell of ABA was all that seemed necessary to propel them onwards and upwards.

So what we didn't fully appreciate – and indeed perhaps no one did when ABA took off in the UK – was that not all autistic children would benefit from or need this type of intensive ABA, and certainly not indefinitely. And that while for some it was a life-changer, enabling them to fulfil their potential, for others it might be a spirit-sapping, soul-destroying intrusion that could have lasting repercussions into adulthood.

In my early enthusiasm, I attributed all resistance to ABA as professional defensiveness, combined with a frequently encountered disdain towards parents. We 'ABA parents' thought the critics were out of touch and patronising. And they in turn thought we were naive and too evangelical. The battle lines around ABA in the UK were thus drawn as a chiefly professional vs parent dispute. It would only be later that I came to hear what autistic people were saying about ABA, and would be required to think again.

10

TreeHouse

In May 1998, after a year of the home programme, we decided the time was right for Danny to join the other children at TreeHouse, a school that had recently opened its doors to its first four pupils: Sonny Carroll, Toby Doré, Chessie Wells and James Hatter.

When I think now about how TreeHouse was started, and my own involvement, what I remember above all is a blur of meetings for over a decade. Finance meetings. Premises meetings. Governing body meetings. Trustee meetings. Staff meetings. Leadership team meetings. Meetings with potential donors. Meetings with interested visitors. Meetings with officials. Meetings with parents.

I wonder how many meetings this book can offer before being consigned to the dustbin. Or how many people I can mention, without that too becoming a list of names that cause you to glaze over.

For there is a long roll call of individuals who should be thanked and credited for doing something remarkable, in being determined, against considerable odds, to establish a new school for autistic children. Not a private school, but one whose places would all be funded as a right (as any other child's would be) by their local authority, and one that would open its doors for years to come to new generations of autistic youngsters. The founding parents I met at my first meeting in 1997 were Karen Edwards (mother of Sonny), Katharine Doré (mother of Toby), Sid Wells (father of Chessie), and Alex and Richard Hatter (parents of James). Determined, delightful, funny, clever – all parents of young, learning-disabled autistic children who couldn't find a local school.

Perhaps I should explain that I came to join them, more by accident than design, because someone at a small speech therapy group told me about these amazing people. That Nick encouraged me to go along to an initial meeting, because – I believe – he felt I needed to meet some like-minded fellow parents and hadn't, at that point, managed to do so. That it would gradually grab his imagination, and that of his family and friends, because they assumed this would be Danny's school (long before the same thing dawned on me). And that having thrown myself in, I would find myself for a brief time as chair of trustees, before gratefully handing it over to Tim Clement-Jones, who would remain at the helm for far longer than he, or any of us, had dared to hope, despite his busy schedule as an eminent lawyer and active member of the House of Lords.

I could tell you about the high-profile launch after which Karen laughingly said 'well we've really got to do it now'. I could tell you about the enormous good fortune in finding some key patrons, such as the mighty Jon Snow, who had been anchor of *Channel 4 News* since 1989.

Or – more significantly, I think – I could tell you about TreeHouse's battle to survive in its early years.

'We're mad, aren't we?' I remember Karen saying at one point, laughing. 'Nobody would try to do this unless they were mad.'

'Can you ever see a time when you might feel like giving up?' I asked.

'No,' she replied. 'Never.'

And that is the point. The stakes were too high, the need too great, to ever give up.

We had to fight, truly. We had to fight to find premises, year after exhausting year. The neighbours in our third temporary accommodation were hostile. Two years later we again nearly faced closure because an inspector decided that our fourth premises (sited on the Coram Family campus) were inadequate for the older pupils – which meant we then had to fight a local planning department that was at first determined to deny planning permission for a fifth, temporary replacement. We weren't safe until we purchased a site in Muswell Hill, where our sixth temporary home was sited, and where we would eventually build our permanent home – all of which involved a hair-raisingly large fundraising effort.

During all of this, we also had to justify our existence on several fronts: to campaigners who hated us because they believed that all special schools should be abolished; to opponents of our chosen approach – ABA, and to many in the SEN world who viewed us with scepticism. Meanwhile, virtually every TreeHouse pupil's place required a costly appeal by their parents (often at tribunal) to access local authority funding.

When I think of the burden we carried it makes me angry. Not just for us but for all the other parents who were going through a similar struggle. From Anna Kennedy, who had to campaign to establish Hillingdon Manor School because there was no alternative for her sons, to the several parents who established ABA schools after TreeHouse, to the parents who felt they had to opt for home-schooling – all these were responses to growing need and an education system failing to keep up.

Local authorities and central government seemed to be oblivious.

The recognised prevalence of autism in the late 1990s was, officially, 4–5 per 10,000 children. But parents could often tell from their own networks that in reality it was far higher. We would later be proved right. In 2000, the Medical Research Council suggested the rate might be 1 per 166, but two years later the NAS's Lorna Wing and David Potter asserted a figure of 1 in 110. More recent figures have quoted one percent, but at the time of writing, some estimates are far higher (US figures cite 1 in 36).[1] Local authority personnel I meet nowadays talk of ever-increasing numbers of children with autism and special educational needs (SEN), while campaigners continue to highlight the deficiencies in the education system, with long waits for diagnosis and appropriate schooling, and high levels of permanent exclusions.

But back in the late 1990s I believed that a short, sharp burst of campaigning might offer a rosier future. Enter Su, my fellow traveller in what would become our joint endeavour to improve education for autistic children.

11

SU AND ELLIOT

It is a mild autumn evening in 1997. I am at home with Danny.

The telephone rings, and a woman introduces herself as Su Thomas.

She has drawn my number from a list on a parent-to-parent helpline.

We start talking and soon realise that we both live in Islington, we both have autistic sons of similar age, and both our boys have accessed special-needs nurseries that are run and funded by our local authority. Su feels Elliot's days at his nursery are numbered, and instead she is planning to set up a home-based ABA programme.

*

The adage that 'one size does not fit all' in autism education was aptly demonstrated by the contrasts between Elliot and Danny. Even though both boys met the diagnostic criteria for autism and learning disability, their differences were far more easily discerned than their similarities.

It was not just that Elliot would dash about while Danny would happily sit for hours; it was their vastly divergent

interests and abilities. Where Danny seemed indifferent to most
toys apart from puzzles, Elliot was a budding builder, engineer
and IT enthusiast. He showed great curiosity about features of
his environment to which Danny seemed oblivious. Shortly
after starting his home programme, Elliot started to speak in
words, then sentences, while Danny (with a few notable excep-
tions, such as 'tss' for 'crisps') remained determinedly loyal to his
favourite phrase: 'oy oy oy'. While mainstream school seemed
out of the question for Danny, it was a highly appropriate goal
for Elliot, whose sunny nature and ability to learn contributed
to his managing well in such a setting, with the right additional
support.

In our early conversations, Su and I also learned about differences between ourselves, despite all that we had in common. Su
grew up in Yorkshire and came to London in her early twenties
to study for an MA at the Royal College of Art. Following a
successful international career in tailoring, she joined the senior
management team at the London College of Fashion, where
she devised the first degree course in menswear.

In the double act that we would become, Su was the glamorous extrovert northerner, expressing Ab Fab flair and
humour along with her big-picture vision to improve the life
chances of autistic children in the UK. Su would say 'we have
to do this' and 'we have to do it now', even though I, the
home-counties boffin, would say 'yes, but …' to many of her
ideas. Su could always be enlisted for any project requiring
taste and visual impact – from designing the layout of a press
release to deciding what I should wear at a conference or
fundraising event. Meanwhile, I would happily prepare, proof-
read and adjust the grammar of draft documents. Su would
keep her wit and hope, however hard things became, and drag
me along when I became lost and dispirited. I learned from
her, as from the TreeHouse founders, that one should seize the
moment and not be afraid.

And so we set off on the next stage of our journeys – joining forces as campaigners and influencers, hoping to change the world. We set up a pressure group under the acronym PACE (Parents Autism Campaign for Education).

12

MARCHING

One night, Nick had a dream that Su and I were taking part in some kind of military parade. After that, the shorthand for the work we were doing – writing letters, meeting people, networking – was 'marching'.

'What have you been doing?' Nick might ask.

'Marching with Su.'

And:

'What are your plans for Saturday morning?'

'Su's coming over, and we're going to do some marching.'

We were hopeful and thought we might be able to bring about some change within a few years. Inevitably, of course, we would discover that the long march of trying to make the world a better place is potentially infinite. But our optimism was warranted, because we were lucky in our connections.

★

This was the era of the recently elected Blair government, and Su's husband was an active member of the Labour Party, with friends in senior positions. And through Nick and his friends, I met Julia Hobsbawm, who with Sarah Macaulay ran one of the hottest, most well-networked PR operations in town. And, as luck would have it, Julia chose to come up to me (it was her initiative, bless her, as if rather than my knocking on her door, she was knocking on mine) and said, 'If there's anything I can do to help …'

First of all, Julia helped Su and me sharpen our campaign message.

We homed in on three broad areas that applied equally – to the potential genius autistic mathematician who would write books and give lectures to thousands, and to the autistic person who throughout their life might struggle to understand what is being said or written, and never acquire the ability to speak.

Here was the birth of PACE's Three Rs campaign for autism education. Instead of the traditional 'reading, 'riting and 'rithmetic', we called for:

Research – to identify how best to help and support autistic children.

Recognition – of autistic children's existence, rights and needs.

Resources – to fund research, more school places and enhanced teacher training.

Julia also helped us devise a high-profile parliamentary launch in May 1999, amidst a wave of publicity. The MP Peter Hain agreed to sponsor a reception in the Jubilee Room at the House of Commons. The room was packed, and several MPs attended.

I had felt jittery about the fact that, cheekily, our launch was on the eve of the National Autistic Society's National Autism Awareness Day, knowing that we might get media coverage that would upstage the NAS's own publicity efforts. Su and Julia were much more robust than I was about this, and pointed out that my desire not to ruffle any feathers would be self-defeating.

'Do you want to launch a high-profile campaign or don't you?' they asked. 'The reason we're doing this is precisely *because* the NAS hasn't done a good enough job at highlighting these vitally important issues.' It was ironic, therefore, and to this day feels unfair, that despite my reticence, and despite Su's leadership and chutzpah, *my* name was primarily linked with the media coverage of the PACE campaign launch. Apparently, our unique selling point was that I was mother of Nick's child – Nick being at the height of his fame as a writer. So it was me who pushed the chief executive of the NAS off a pre-arranged slot on the daily BBC TV programme *The Vanessa Show*. Instead of Paul Cann, there was I – on live TV – talking about Danny and the Three Rs campaign.

At the back of my mind, while all this was happening, I was thinking 'This is surreal', and wondering if there was any way at all that it would eventually translate into a better deal for autistic children and their families. You can appear on live TV, watched by millions, talk about a cause, and then what? Has anything changed? That is what I was thinking later, when the adrenalin had left me and I was picking Danny up from school, and it is sometimes what I still think.

Except, in the long run, perhaps the most sustainable of our achievements at that point was to galvanise the NAS into establishing a campaigns, policy and communications team. A team that would, in due course, be instrumental in the passing of the first ever condition-specific legislation in the UK – the Autism Act of 2009.[1]

But it is only many years later, when I look back, that I can see the obvious glaring omission in all of this. When I refer to those attending the launch of the Three Rs campaign, do I mention anyone there who is autistic? Did it even occur to us that autistic people should be among the invitees? Or have a say in what kind of educational provision would have most suited their needs and for which, therefore, we should be calling? Admittedly, we were focused on children and early intervention, so perhaps we were off the hook somewhat; parents are on the whole considered legitimate spokespeople for their children's rights and needs. But the fact is, I'm not sure if it even dawned on us.

It was, to all intents and purposes, an event about autism to which no autistic person was invited. Later I would come to hold the phrase 'nothing about us without us' – a cornerstone of the disability rights movement – as a moral imperative. But at the time, none of this entered my head. We were simply trying to help improve things for children who were unable to speak for themselves. Not such a bad thing really, but not – it has to be said – fully informed by all the arguments that in reality surround the whole contested terrain of autism education, autism representation, autism campaigning. The things I would learn, from the people I would subsequently meet, will come later. A mountain climb awaited us, and in summer 1999 we were still in the foothills.

Part 3

SOLIDARITY AND CONFLICT

'The culture of science makes us believe that medicine and psychology can tell us truths about our bodies, when in fact they can only tell us about the particular set of phenomena we're looking at, or more precisely, about what our time and culture tell us is meaningful to look at.'

Roy Richard Grinker, *Isabel's World*

I believe few conditions come close to autism in terms of the divisions and controversies to which it gives rise. Differences of opinion about the fundamental nature of autism persist. Is it a contrivance built upon the arbitrary elision of particular behaviours with no biological underpinning, or will scientists one day be able to identify a unifying set of molecular attributes? Is it a disease, a disorder or just a different way of being? These differences lead to contrasting perspectives on how best to support autistic people, and who to listen to when seeking support. There are multiple 'camps' and conflicts, offering up different heroes and villains – parents, doctors, drug companies, advocates of different therapies and autistic people with different standpoints on their own condition and on the kind of support they want.

In the middle of this battleground, Danny and I journeyed on, confronting personal challenges that interweaved with the bigger themes of the time, and meeting new people who inspired and befriended us.

13

DONNA, DANIEL AND PAUL

I am at a meeting for parents in Islington whose children have recently been diagnosed with autism. This is before ABA, before TreeHouse, before campaigning. I am dutifully attending the group, even though I am getting nothing from being there, except to notice Donna, and to like her.

Donna is a small, round woman with streaks of burgundy and crimson in her hair. She has an infectious laugh and she talks nineteen to the dozen. Her son Daniel is nearly three years old, has a mop of thick, straw-coloured hair and is a little angel, quietly lining up trains while Donna talks with the group.

I will later be told by Paul, Daniel's dad, that in his early years Daniel screamed all day, every day. The screaming persisted for several months after a colossal seizure had diverted him from a typical developmental path onto a different trajectory heading somewhere new and initially foreign. He had been talking in four-word sentences, he had been interacting happily with his large extended family. Then wham. Shutdown. His seizure was a feature of a rare form of epilepsy called Landau Kleffner, and the autism seemed to come along as an integral fellow traveller.

The screaming had stopped by the time Donna and Daniel came to the support group, and my recollection was that he was quiet, gentle and docile throughout the meeting, while Donna spoke of the double whammy of Landau Kleffner and autism.

I thought we had little in common, until I found out that Donna and Daniel lived around the corner from me in a council property directly facing the Lower East Stand of Highbury Stadium. (This was not ideal for Paul, a lifelong Tottenham supporter.) About a year after our first meeting, aware that Donna and Paul had recently been advised to start exploring appropriate educational provision for Daniel, I invited her to come and observe the final workshop being organised as part of Danny's ABA home programme. I did not know at the time how overwhelming this invitation was for Donna. She had to come into a strange house, the home of someone she hardly knew, and to meet not just Danny (no problem at all meeting him), but also the ABA consultant, Nick and all Danny's tutors.

Quite soon she left, and later reported to Paul that we were an awful bunch of middle-class people who seemed unable to accept that our child was disabled. After that we had no contact for a while, but everything would change because of TreeHouse.

★

Having read about TreeHouse in the local paper, Donna and Paul arranged a visit, from which they went away determined that this would be Daniel's school. They liked the family ethos, the fact that it was (temporarily) in a townhouse, which made it feel more homely and less institutional than the other schools and nurseries they had seen. They liked the continuous stream of positivity, the atmosphere of hope and belief, the smiles of the teaching staff and the unusually low levels of crying and distress.

Donna and Paul were new to the whole sorry process of SEN. They were astonished that none of the local professionals had suggested they visit TreeHouse, nor even mentioned it. Donna was furious that people who did not know their boy, who had never even met him, were empowered to make decisions about his future, ostensibly on the grounds of need but in reality, chiefly on grounds of cost.

This is such a well-worn path, for so many families.[1] Suffice it to say that, finally, after various conversations and negotiations, on and off the record, threats of tribunal and so on, Daniel became the next pupil to start at TreeHouse. With his mischievous smile and big personality, he immediately won everyone's hearts, just as Donna and Paul were instantly appreciated among the staff and TreeHouse families for their warmth and sincerity.

Out of school, our families grew closer. The closeness was punctuated with some joint outings, in particular to funfairs. The Christmas indoor fair at Olympia saw the two boys and me sharing a mini-roller-coaster ride, positioned at the head of the dragon to get maximum effect as we plunged through the water in the dip, both Dans shrieking with pleasure and all three of us emerging soaked but triumphant. Both boys adored the sensations and were totally fearless. The din of machinery and music and people screaming with excitement and terror, the spectacle of colour and patterns and outsize adult cartoons decorating the rides everywhere you look, the kids and the toddlers and the grown-ups crowding round – it's enough of an assault on anyone's senses, but our Dans were transported with pleasure. And of course, I need to add that for many autistic people, this battering of the senses would be a living hell, as it was for Toby when he and Katharine attempted a similar outing with us a few weeks later.

Donna came to some of the girls' nights out that a group of us organised – trips into the West End to dance, like we didn't have a care in the world – a giant, defiant V-sign to all the battles we were fighting, and an escape from the more usual causes of broken nights due to our children's sleep issues.

And occasionally there would be long telephone conversations with Donna, which I so wish I had recorded and transcribed so that I could share with you all her wit and originality and wisdom. Streams of consciousness darting all over the place, several threads running concurrently with pauses for laughter or exclamation, penetrating questions about everything but no time for an answer before the next topic rushed in …

Over the years I learned that Donna had been born with hydrocephaly, necessitating a shunt (drainage tube) from the brain into the lymph system in the neck and causing, in her own words, her learning difficulties and volatile moods. At birth, her insides were located in unusual parts of her abdomen, necessitating several operations to reposition them. In her teenage years, after a particularly bad experience she wound up in a women's refuge. Unsurprisingly, she mistrusted men. But Paul was different. He had always been a friend, and he was someone she thought of so highly that she had tried to matchmake him with one of her best friends. It took a long time for Paul to pluck up the courage to say that actually, it was her, Donna, with whom he'd been in love, for years.

Paul is a very big man, resembling a larger-than-life Ray Winstone, with fairer hair and a gentler demeanour, but they could be cousins or brothers in terms of their facial features and their voices. Donna and Paul lived apart and their relationship would remain permanently ambiguous. He had his own place in East London, but would often be needed to help with childcare back in Highbury.

Whatever the highs and lows of their chequered time together, they had three lovely children. Daniel would have two younger sisters, Jamey and Billie. Donna cherished all three as miracles, and in a later time, when she became a born-again Christian, they were specifically God's miracles. Paul could not share her belief in the Divine, but this difference of outlook did not encumber their joint parental endeavour. And, unlike some fathers of disabled children, he was in for the long haul, and destined to be one of this book's heroes.

14

THE MMR CONTROVERSY

Conversations with Donna and Paul rarely go the way of small talk. They steer inexorably back to the big things, the profound underpinning forces of love, life, death.

Early in our friendship, I would discuss with both Donna and Paul the arguments around whether autism is a condition that can or should be cured, or whether it is more like a fundamental feature of someone's identity, their selfhood. We were at the height of the MMR controversy. Newspapers and TV and the internet were all buzzing with tales of children going into autistic regression at around eighteen months old, after having received the first dose of the jab to immunise against Measles, Mumps and Rubella. Most health experts said that the MMR vaccine posed no risk, while a small group of doctors and alternative therapists said that it did. Families were split on the issue, so that any decision to administer, or refrain from, the MMR vaccination could be attacked as irresponsible, as a wilful disregard of evidence, or both.

The controversy originated at the Royal Free Hospital, where Andrew Wakefield had been employed as a research fellow, and from where, in 1998, he published his now notorious paper in *The Lancet*.[1] This paper, co-authored by colleagues of his at the

Royal Free, told of a group of children whose dual autistic and gastrointestinal (GI) symptoms seemed to have emerged after having been administered the MMR jab at around eighteen months. A group of parents (encouraged by Wakefield) embarked on a class-action lawsuit to try to sue the drug companies whom they held responsible. As all good scientists know, correlation does not equal causation, but there were many parents who felt it was indeed the jab that had caused their child's new symptoms.[2]

At a press conference in 1998, Wakefield went further than colleagues had anticipated or intended. He expressed the view that the MMR immunisation should be withdrawn while further investigation took place.

I wonder sometimes if he ever looks back and speculates how life might have been, not just for him, but for all those who would be drawn into the endless machinations, character assassinations, claims and counterclaims, all the far-reaching and long-term ramifications of his assertion, if he had kept his mouth shut.

But he didn't. Instead, he went on speaking and writing and campaigning and networking and proclaiming the rightness of his cause with such fervour that a kind of collective hysteria ensued in much of the Western world. Wave upon wave of polemical writing, conferences, TV dramatisations and character assassinations followed. Congressional hearings took place in the USA. Death threats, trolling, conspiracy theories abounded. The conflict was not simply about whether or not MMR might have triggered autism in a group of young children. It became a cause about vaccinations in toto, one in which expressions of concern about public health were assumed to be a mere front for the profiteering pharmaceutical companies, and – on the other hand – where the actions of Wakefield and his supporters were viewed with dismay, because of the fear that they would lead to unnecessarily high levels of avoidable illness and even death.

Wakefield became a messianic figure in some circles.

'I believe Andrew Wakefield is our saviour,' wrote one believer on a parents e-group.

'From what [I might have responded] do you think he's saving you?'

Perhaps her need for a hero was rooted in the fact that until this doctor had made autism a prominent issue in the media, no one had listened to her and taken her or her child's condition seriously. No one had come forward to help or truly understand. Speech therapists and social workers and psychologists had conducted endless repetitive assessments but had failed to follow through with tangible assistance. Or perhaps she was traumatised by her child's disability and looked for heroes and villains to convert her rage and grief into a battle of good and evil. Here, at last, was a charismatic doctor who believed – when no one else did – that her child's gastrointestinal symptoms were real. A man who, moreover, was prepared – like David against Goliath – to take on the pharma and public health establishment for the sake of vulnerable children who were too often overlooked.

Later, I would meet some of the protagonists in the debate and hear more about their points of view. I was not immediately prepared to dismiss the conviction of parents, even while I was aware that the occurrence of autistic regression at eighteen months had been noted long before the introduction of MMR.

But still, Donna, Paul and I responded to the furore with a profound unease. Not so much at the claims about cause and evidence, but at the underlying message coming from the anti-vaxxers. The message was that autism was one of the worst things that could happen to a person, a lot worse than having measles-related complications. Autism was described by some as if it was an evil monster lurking in the wings waiting to seize young children and destroy their essence.

This simply didn't wash with us; we didn't feel our autistic boys were thus afflicted. For all the times when they seemed distressed, there were other times when they were clearly happy. They derived pleasure in many things. They were our Dans, in all their newly apparent, autistic, Dan-ness.

It probably took us a little while to arrive at this place of peace and acceptance. Early on in Danny's life I had wanted to find answers for why he had a left-sided weakness, and what had caused it. But soon this curiosity abated, as Danny came fully into view as a whole and adorable person, not a damaged one. So it saddened Donna, Paul and me to note that some other parents seemed to get stuck in an initial state of shock and sadness. While we understood and empathised with an initial shock, and sense of loss, we were concerned for those parents who seemed to go on feeling bitter and resentful, stuck in a PTSD-type state, five, ten, fifteen years later – as if all along life had owed them a different child.

It would be many years before I came to appreciate fully what damage unfiltered expressions of parental yearning can do to the autistic person's self-esteem, and the anger felt by some autistic adults as a result of what they experienced as deep rejection. It would explain why parents and scientists who sought to cure autism were vilified as 'curebies' and regarded as the enemy.

But back in those early days it was Paul who summed it up beautifully, when discussing the goal of curing autism: 'It's like putting your child up for adoption, and then asking for another person's child in their place.' Adding: 'People would be horri-fied if you did that.'

Many years later, I would approach these issues from the perspective of moral philosophy and medical ethics. My thoughts would turn to whether it is morally right to seek to prevent autism. But the opportunity to explore these ideas in any depth would have to wait for several years.

Instead, after the initial concerns and readjustments, we didn't want to spend our days thinking about why our Dans were as they were. Rather, we wanted to help them be all they could be. We wanted them to flourish and to have fun, to be well and pain-free. The battle to achieve this last goal would turn out to be much harder than we anticipated. Happily, we didn't know this at the time. The fun bit was, mercifully, not only easy but also infectious and life-affirming. We were sharing a big adventure.

Even so, some debates cannot be shut down, or circumnavigated. They have to be faced head on. Despite my reluctance to get involved, either for or against the MMR vaccination, I unwittingly became entangled in the drama surrounding it.

★

Drs X and Y were high-profile protagonists occupying polar-opposite positions in the MMR debate. I had met each of them, in different contexts, and each seemed to think that I might be able to help them. They both chose to contact me over the period of a few weeks.

They were looking for dirt.

'What do you know about Dr Y?' asked Dr X.

'Is there anything you can tell me about Dr X?' asked Dr Y.

I could have said quite a lot. Or I could have told them to back off. 'I am just Danny's mum. It's the weekend. Leave me alone.'

Instead, I told each that the other one seemed to be a nice person, and that I didn't know enough about the scientific foundations of their arguments to say anything more. Which is true. I quite liked them both. I did not consider either of them to be bad people. But in retrospect, perhaps I should have given them a piece of my mind and asked them to stop – as I perceived it – relishing the battle, getting off on the adrenalin of conflict, to stop behaving like angry missile-throwing children with points to prove and egos to feed, and to start promoting a calm discussion like grown-ups.

And this reveals one of the dilemmas I have faced when writing the book. Am I too enamoured of my characters to reveal their uglier sides? Is everyone I talk about too relentlessly nice? And is it tedious for the reader to plough through a tale in which the characters are – if not saintly, then at least likeable or virtuous in some way?

The thing is this: the autism world is jam-packed with hostility and resentment, with attempts to capsize careers and undermine opposing standpoints* – even within a movement that ostensibly celebrates diversity! I don't want to go there. And at a personal level, there is enough anger in me with regard to the wider forces of indifference and under-provision, of cruel practice and institutional abuse. Why would I want to deplete my energies further, with profligate personal animus?

Gratitude, in contrast, is constituted differently. It generates hope and momentum, and shines a light in places and on people that might otherwise be overlooked. And it is in this spirit that I choose now to write about another person who played a role – not just in the MMR debate, but also closer to home – in the story of Danny and me.

---

* One of the debates I find particularly unhelpful is the retrospective exploration of Kanner and Asperger as if they are in competition, as if one of them is the true pioneer and one of them is the chief culprit (be this in relation to diagnostic validity or Nazi collaboration).

15

MMR and Simon Murch

Danny's first year at TreeHouse had gone well.

He was happy to go there each day, and – defying the clichéd view of non-verbal, learning-disabled autistic children who will be forever alone and unable to connect – he and Toby (son of founding parent Katharine) forged an indelible friendship. They would hug one another spontaneously, engage in tentative and then intense eye contact, and express themselves through unique vocalisations. This friendship has sustained over the years, even when, as adults, they have lived in different countries from one another and can meet only infrequently.

Despite these developments at TreeHouse, Nick and I were increasingly concerned about Danny's physical well-being. His place at TreeHouse was secure, and he had adapted well following our formal separation. We had managed to find a routine that enabled him to have quality time with each parent, and we in turn were able to get some nights of undisturbed sleep and time to see our respective friends in the reassuring knowledge that Danny was happy and secure in both our homes.

What we were not coping well with, though, was the fact that Danny experienced frequent episodes of pain. He couldn't tell us directly, but his tears and screams and sudden doubling-up were eloquent enough. He also couldn't tell us where the pain resided, but careful observation and data-gathering informed us that it correlated with chronic constipation, occasional over-flow that seemed like diarrhoea, and general discomfort and distress after meals and before opening his bowels.

This, as I started to recall, had been a feature of his early life, something we hoped had been dealt with by the surgery to repair his inguinal hernias when he was a baby. But as Danny approached his seventh birthday, it was becoming clear that we could no longer wish it away, or try to diminish its significance. Our GP readily agreed to a referral to a local hospital that specialised in paediatric gastroenterology, and one that had several young patients with autism. The Royal Free.

★

The extent of the standoff between different 'camps' at the Royal Free quickly became apparent.

In their readiness to discount Wakefield's assertion, many medics were keen to dismiss any appearance of GI disorder in autistic children. After all, until then it was chiefly Wakefield who had postulated any link between autism and GI problems, and he – they thought – was a charlatan. And wasn't autism primarily a psychological condition?

The doctor we encountered first was probably a member of this anti-Wakefield camp. He appeared uninterested to the point of hostility when Nick and I tried to explain the severity of Danny's pain-related distress. I may not be right in recalling that he rolled his eyes, but the memory is crystal clear of him saying dismissively and with boredom: 'Autistic children cry a lot.'

That's all he said.

'But,' we tried to say, 'when he's not in pain, Danny is a sunny, placid, happy person who rarely cries. He's sociable and enjoys so much of his life. He's cooperative and gentle and has a great sense of humour. The pain seems to come from nowhere – no external triggers. It can happen at different times of day, in different places, with different people. It's *real physical pain.*'

Yet it felt like an impossible task to convince this doctor. I would later learn that this tendency to attribute everything to Danny's autism and learning disability, rather than to take seriously the possibility of a distinct underlying medical problem, has an official name: diagnostic overshadowing. It means that doctors fail to be curious about symptoms that they would take seriously in a neurotypical person, assuming that the disability explains everything.

Danny had no speech; he couldn't let us know through language what he was going through, he couldn't gesture to the source of the pain. He made no connection with the question 'Where does it hurt?' or with the picture we showed him of a body, in the hope he could point to the corresponding offending area. And the physical signs upon examination were unrevealing. His tummy was soft and he didn't flinch at the points where slight pressure was exerted.

'I wonder if the doctor thinks we're making it up,' I said to Nick later.

Was I? Was I over-dramatising something? Was I over-influenced by other parents who told stories of GI problems in their autistic children? Was I trying to get on a bandwagon? When Danny was happy, and the immediacy of his joy seemed to banish all concern for his health, a small voice in my head posed such questions, and additional ones: am I a crap mother? Am I trying to prove something through Danny?

To add to our disquiet, new rumours started to circulate about parents of autistic children, as if we were back in the world of refrigerator mothers. Bettelheim's accusation that autism was caused by cold, unresponsive parents had now mutated into a new form of parent-blaming: namely, that parents were convincing themselves that their children were physically unwell because this was easier to deal with than a psychological condition, or an inherited personality feature.

Munchausen Syndrome by Proxy (MSbP)* reared its head as an accusation frequently levelled at parents, especially mothers. It would evolve into Fabricated or Induced Illness (FII) over the years.[1] At heart, here was an idea that parents met their emotional needs through inventing pathology in their children.

Yet the moment Danny's pain behaviour returned, any such self-questioning went out the window. Instead of beating myself up in case I was an MSbP mum, I beat myself up for failing to make a strong enough case about Danny's distress to the doctors. I would pour out my despair and anger in long streams of consciousness at the computer, but I never sent them on in raw form, because angry and desperate mothers sometimes alienate the very professionals on whom their children depend.

The first doctor pretty much sent us away. So on the next occasion we asked to see Simon Murch, one of the co-authors of the original Wakefield article, and who had recently been promoted to the status of consultant.

The contrast could not have been more startling. His team were attentive and sympathetic, and took us seriously.

Because Danny's pain had been escalating, we were more than willing for him to undergo an investigative procedure. In fact, we were desperate to find out why Danny was having so much trouble with regard to the whole business of getting food into, and waste out of, his body. We didn't want him to go through his life so often crying, so often stopping in his tracks and doubling over, emitting agonised shrieks and sometimes spending whole days in torment.

Finally, in 2001, Simon Murch felt it would be appropriate to conduct an endoscopy and colonoscopy, to see if there were any

---

*   MSbP is also known as Factitious Disorder Imposed on Another (FDIA).

abnormalities that might explain Danny's distress. We were relieved and full of hope that something would be discovered that could help him.

As it turned out, nothing untoward was found – no signs of inflammation, no ulcers. Yet Danny seemed a whole lot better just from the experience of a massive pre-operative clearance of his intestines. We weren't aware at the time how revealing this would be about the underlying problems with Danny's gut. Nor were we aware how much pressure Simon was under, on the one hand from the medical establishment for his association with the original *Lancet* article, and on the other hand from those who continued to believe and espouse the MMR theory. All we knew at our first meetings with Simon was that he was Danny's concerned, cautious, gentle doctor.

I also appreciated an integrity I had already observed in Simon at a conference I attended before he became Danny's doctor.[2] Simon said clearly, in the presence of Andrew Wakefield and the audience who overwhelmingly hailed Wakefield as a hero: 'I am being told that there is likely to be a measles outbreak in North London.'

And then the magic words: 'I don't know what to do.'

Not many people in the audience seemed to appreciate this. That he was going through an inner turmoil about whether he should publicly break ranks with Wakefield and be accused of betrayal. Simon had his own hypotheses about why some autistic children presented with GI problems, and he did not consider that the measles virus was the culprit.

But I loved his honesty, particularly in front of an audience who would not welcome it.

In all the years of my involvement with autism, I have liked best those people who humbly admit to how much they don't know.

Later, Simon would leave the Royal Free (much to our sadness) and everything would spill out into the public domain.

In 2003, he wrote a letter to *The Lancet* refuting any MMR–autism link, and a public disagreement between Simon and Wakefield featured on BBC radio and was reported in national newspapers.[3]

Despite this, he would still be dragged through the mire, thanks to a General Medical Council (GMC) hearing that was launched following a series of reports by the journalist Brian Deer. The allegation would be that he behaved unethically by subjecting young autistic children to unnecessary interventions. Nick and I were, and still are, puzzled as to why Deer was intent on pursuing what seemed like a vindictive line of inquiry against Simon – a practising clinician and academic in a field crying out for more work, and someone who was now entirely distanced from the anti-MMR-vaccine lobby.

After one of the longest investigations in GMC history, he was finally cleared.

For Nick and me, the irony of the allegation was only too clear. We had been desperate for investigative procedures that might shed light on what Danny was going through. In contrast to Deer's charge of recklessness, it was Simon's caution that had been so evident when treating Danny.

16

COREY

We were still in the dark about what was afflicting Danny and would continue to be so for years. To thrive against this background of physical pain has been the struggle of his life, and – indirectly – of mine. I would later say it made autism and learning disability, setting up a school and a pressure group, seem straightforward in comparison.

To illustrate the extent of my preoccupation with Danny's ill health, I recall a conversation with a friend who rang me one weekend afternoon.

'It's happened to us,' he said.

'What? What's happened?'

'The thing that happens to so many parents who have an autistic child …'

Oh no, I thought. Poor things. He's phoning to tell me that his son, like ours, has started to suffer this dreadful GI pain. Poor, poor things.

But instead, he said:

'A and I are getting divorced.'

And my inner reaction was one of relief. I didn't actually say, 'Oh *that*! Phew, I thought it was something much worse', but it's pretty much what I felt.

In retrospect, two observations stand out.

The first is the extent to which – in my mind – the possibility of the child's pain and the parents' own well-being seemed inextricably intertwined. *'It's happened to us'* recalls families' sense of being 'disabled by association' when they have a disabled child. The battles and the isolation ripple out in ways that affect all who are close. Families lose friends, miss out on activities that others take for granted, feel disconnected and abandoned because some of the challenges they face are so different from those of other families. I have felt this in relation to Danny's disability, up to a point, but I have known it to a far greater extent in relation to Danny's gastrointestinal illness. 'Normal' life, 'normal' enjoyments, 'normal' achievements, all seem to be experienced through a filter, like the Lady of Shalott looking at the landscape only through a mirror. The barrier of the sorrow of Danny's pain has sometimes muffled everything.

The second observation is my friend's assumption that divorce is all but inevitable if you have an autistic child. Indeed, a commonly quoted statistic was that eighty percent of these marriages break up. This figure, as well as the implication that autism somehow destroys relationships, would be roundly debunked in an important article published in 2013.[1] But it continues in some quarters as a belief to this day. Certainly there are added pressures – ones that Nick and I both experienced in Danny's first few years, and which probably underscored the differences between us that predated his birth. But we could equally claim that Danny's disability then enabled us, post-divorce, to focus our attention on him, rather than on battles with one another; to remain in continual and cordial dialogue about Danny and his medical problems, and then in time to acquire the reinforcements (step-parents, new siblings) that we all needed.

I was probably feeling particularly dismissive about the downside of divorce at the time my friend phoned me, because by then Nick's partner Amanda was proving herself to be an indefatigable and welcome addition to the extended family. This no doubt contributed to my view that, for all its earlier traumas, divorce seemed to me so much the lesser challenge compared with having a child who suffers from recurrent pain – particularly a pain that the medical profession seem helpless to alleviate.

That conversation was a litmus test for the devastation that Danny's illness wrought. It also serves as a foundation stone for the solidarity, empathy and respect with which I hold all parents whose children are chronically unwell.

I sometimes wondered if I should abandon campaigning for education, and instead focus entirely on the biomedical issues that seemed to impact so strongly on Danny. Yet I knew that while GI problems affected some children with autism, the challenge to improve the education system affected all. The evidence that GI problems were a minority interest was all around me. There was Elliot, bursting with physical health. There was Daniel, his epilepsy controlled well through medication, getting through life seemingly pain-free, and look at Sonny, Toby and Chessie and all the kids in the TreeHouse playground. Listen to their parents. A minority reported GI problems, but, thankfully, the majority did not.

In any case, while I felt helpless in relation to Danny's illness, I believed that TreeHouse and PACE were actively helpful, and that we had a chance to make things better for many. However much Danny's physical problems were affecting our family, there was a wider, more universal need that still merited attention. Things would have to get worse before I finally withdrew from the world of autism education and campaigning.

So onwards we went. And it was during these years that a crucial recruit to Danny's band of angels arrived. Without whom, there simply could not have been any more story. Danny and I would have sunk. Corey was as crucial as that.

★

It is a sunny afternoon in midsummer. The trees that line our road are in full bloom, as Danny and I drive home from school.

A young man in his mid-twenties is walking along the pavement. He opens the gate and goes up to our front door. As I pull in and park, he turns round and smiles at us.

My recollection is of love at first sight – platonic, no, more like *familial* love. How do I know, even at this precise moment, that here is someone we need, and who perhaps in his own unique way also needs us?

Heaven knows. But it is as if I do know, in my very soul, that an angel has arrived. He is of slight build, attractive, kind-looking, with light auburn hair and a gentle aura. He explains that Su has suggested he visit us, because he is interested in working with autistic children, having recently completed a psychology degree and having already met Elliot.

We go into the house together, sit and chat, while Corey and Danny grow accustomed to one another. And in that first conversation I ask Corey if he would be willing to work with Danny after school. Corey is surprised. What about references? Might I not need them? What about seeing his CV? What about a more formal interview process?

Corey, I can see already that you and Danny have formed a connection. I have never known anything quite as clearly as I know right now that you are the person we have been waiting for.

What I didn't yet know was this:

Corey, you will be there in our best and our worst times. In due course you will come and live with us for a few years. You will be there night and day when Danny is desperately unwell, and you will cherish him as if he were your younger brother. And Danny, for his part, will love you as his big brother, mentor, teacher, protector, warrior, defender. With you, Danny and I will laugh and have fun, be brave and enjoy many adventures. With you we will go to the seaside, to funfairs, to concerts and films, we will travel in trains and boats and planes, and – oh heaven – we will go to Las Vegas to see Cirque du Soleil perform the Beatles' Love album. Danny will have the honour of being your best man when you get married. With you, he will be granted courage to face things that no one should have to face. And thanks to your intrepid and loyal soul, I will be given the strength to endure, and to find hope.

Corey started working with Danny almost immediately and has never left our lives.

17

FOUR PRAYERS

It's 2003. Another autumn, and the days are drawing in.

There are four things I have been praying will happen for the sake of TreeHouse's future, and it seems that each depends upon the others.

The first is that an impending charity event will help us raise significant funds for our work.

The second is that TreeHouse will attract a head teacher whose presence will reassure staff, parents and local authorities that here is a school that serves its pupils well.

The third prayer is that Haringey Council will grant planning permission, so that our plans to develop a national centre on the Muswell Hill site we are poised to purchase might at last come to fruition.

And the fourth is that somehow, all will work out for J – one of our pupils – and his family.

The fate of all these prayers will be sealed during one epic week in October 2003, on (as I recall) Monday, Wednesday and Friday.

The interdependence is terrifying. It feels as if TreeHouse will only survive if all four endeavours are successful. For it is unlikely that Gill Bierschenk, our hoped-for head, will be willing to take the job unless Haringey grant planning permission and hence a secure future for the school.

Yet planning permission is unlikely to be granted unless Haringey's SEN department supports TreeHouse's application. And unfortunately, for the last few months, TreeHouse has got itself in a terrible mess with J, a pupil from Haringey. We have tried to meet his needs, but he needs more space, he needs specialists with more experience than our in-house staff have yet acquired, he needs a greater repertoire of strategies than we have at our disposal, and our communication with his parents has been inadequate.

The fundraising dinner is the first event of this fateful week. We dress up in our finery, Nick speaks, the well-known autism specialist Simon Baron-Cohen speaks, and then the auctioneer gets cracking. He has an autistic nephew, and I know the family, which is no doubt another piece of luck for us. His passion and cajoling during the auction mean that we raise a substantial six-figure sum – far bigger than we had expected. This is fantastic. It means that, as long as everything else turns out OK later in the week, we will be able to consolidate the work of the school and the charity, and help many more children over the coming years.

Two days later, we sit in a committee room in Haringey Council. Several supporters are in attendance. Here are our architects and our planning advisers; here is Gill, our hoped-for head teacher, sitting with the head of Haringey's SEN department. Joining them are the head teachers of the two local primary schools that will be adjacent to TreeHouse if the permission goes ahead. And here are several TreeHouse families, including the family of J, to offer encouragement.

The meeting itself is almost anticlimactic in contrast to the high tension we had experienced with Camden's planning department. Certainly, we have done everything by the book, visiting councillors, organising local consultation events, leafleting the neighbourhood. But still we cannot be sure, after the previous planning battles, that all this will pay off.

We needn't have feared. There are no obstructions, only words of support – including, crucially, from the head of the SEN department, who knows us warts and all.

The decision is made quickly and the committee chair says simply: 'Welcome to Haringey.'

As easy as that.

No final, last-minute twists, no eleventh-hour cliffhangers.

Welcome to Haringey.

At last.

★

This should have been intoxicating stuff. We could now be certain that Gill would be our long-awaited head, we knew that our agonising search for a permanent home was over and we knew we could put flesh on our aspirations to be a charity with national influence. I remember the warm congratulations and excitement radiating from our planning team, the local education officials, the families, at the celebratory drinks. In retrospect I can truly feel the pleasure and the relief at this extraordinary landmark evening. But not at the time.

As I stood and smiled and chatted in that bar, what I was feeling was neither triumphant nor happy. All I felt was sadness and dread, which I had to disguise for all I was worth because the reason for the undertow was confidential. What only a handful of us knew, during that evening of celebration in the pub, was that within two days we would be delivering a hammer blow to J's parents.

J could no longer stay at TreeHouse.

Beneath this stark message lay an ocean of distress, as well as a whole litany of accusations that were levelled against us, and some private and emotional discussions with J's parents. I had been utterly torn as vice-chair of trustees. We didn't set up TreeHouse to fail children and parents, but it felt to me at the time that this is what we had done in J's case.

In hindsight it is clear that J needed something more than TreeHouse could deliver at that stage of its development, but I wasn't thinking of it in those measured terms at the time. Instead, it felt like a catastrophe.

18

Depression and Identity

The stress of the previous few months, including some difficult events at home (Danny and I had moved house – positive yet exhausting; a cousin had died suddenly; Ingrid had breast cancer and her impending mastectomy loomed on the horizon; Danny was often unwell) – all of these things meant I was at a low ebb. So, unsurprisingly I guess, that final meeting in that epic week tipped my brain chemistry into meltdown.

There was no joy or hope linked to the achievements of the week. Only despair, guilt, doubt, anguish and a terrible fear that everything we had been working towards was somehow tainted and misguided. All this, with a growing dark sadness about J and his family, which instead of loosening its grip, dragged me down and down over the ensuing weeks.

I couldn't read. I couldn't write.

I couldn't make phone calls.

It would take me a day to decipher an email. It would take me another day to find the energy to transfer wet clothes and towels from the washing machine to dry on the radiators. After which I would collapse and stare into the middle distance, or lie in bed, thinking about nothing, but all the time feeling a spiritual pain that paralysed me.

Sometimes I would cry and cry, and other times even tears took too much energy, and I retreated into a blank – yet still painful – space.

I fantasised about suicide as something longed-for and wonderful, what Andrew Solomon has called its 'siren call'.[1]

What do I want to say about all of this now? I certainly don't want to milk it for sympathy. Given what J and his family were facing – no TreeHouse, the prospect that he would have to leave home to attend a residential school once a place could be found, and in the interim would retreat into a place of torment that his mother M would describe later as a deep regression – there is no competition for trauma.

Instead, I want to offer some of what I learned over the next few months. Although I could barely think, there were a few cognitive faculties still at work, and they in turn converted what I was going through into thoughts about illness and the power of love. Those months of despair also influenced how I would later come to view autism itself.

*

During the slow recovery period, I managed to read Lewis Wolpert's *Malignant Sadness*.[2] And I seized upon the suggestion that, among the various triggers that can cause depression, lies 'the loss of a cherished idea'. And yes, it seemed as if all the hope and belief I had invested in TreeHouse had come crashing down. Were we a sham operation? Were we doing more harm than good? Had we, in our TreeHouse endeavour, created a monster? I had no belief left, and assumed that more catastrophes were about to occur, that the story of J and his parents was just the start.

These fears haunted me, but there was one truth that got me through. Not an idea or a concept or a belief, but a powerful energy coming from a different part of my self. It was love of

Danny. Despite all the self-doubt and longing not to be anymore, there was enough rationality to recognise that, however awful I was or felt, *Danny would not be better off without me.*

It was Danny's presence in my life that got me up in the morning and enabled me to make his breakfast, dress him, drive him to school. When home again I would collapse for hours. Nick had learned to drive in order to help with the school run, and Paul also offered his services so that the two Dans could travel together. Corey or another helper would then be there to keep Danny safe and entertained until suppertime. And somehow, because evenings were slightly less agonising than mornings and afternoons, I could still cook Danny's supper, run his bath, sing to him, carry him up to bed at night and tell him wholeheartedly how much I loved him. Each morning was like having to climb the same mountain over and over again. But we hung on in there, Danny and I, until the antidepressants had time to work.

So this is what held me up. 1 Corinthians 13.[3] When faith and hope are gone, there can still be love. At times like these, love is all there is, the only thing between death and life.

*

Living with depression like this required me to examine from a new angle the vexed domain of mental health and mental illness, the overlapping issues of identity and selfhood, and the role of medication.

In the throes of it, I came to know with total conviction that depression was a state of ill health, rather than merely feeling fed up, sad, melancholic. I knew I needed help and had no fears about taking higher doses of medication. I didn't care about the things that some people wonder about – that drugs might alter my essence, take away my identity or selfhood. Rather, I considered that it was the depression that was altering me, taking me away from the person I 'truly' am, and that chemicals – perhaps like insulin for a diabetic – would bring about homeostasis, equilibrium, balance.

In any case, my identity mattered not a jot. When you're in such pain, when every second of your life feels like you might not be able to bear it, who cares if some drug changes who you are? You'll do anything, anything, just to take the pain away.

What alarms me about this is the knowledge that I would be terrible under torture. I would give away all manner of secrets in a jiffy.

★

This period of depression also influenced my views about autism.

Two reflections emerged.

The first concerns the relationship between depression, autism and identity.

Powerful testimonies by autistic people assert autism as an identity. For example, Jim Sinclair's crucial essay 'Don't Mourn for Us' includes the following:

> Autism isn't something a person *has*, or a 'shell' that a person is trapped inside. There's no normal child hidden behind the autism. Autism is a way of being. It is *pervasive*; it colors every experience, every sensation, perception, thought, emotion, and encounter, every aspect of existence. It is not possible to separate the autism from the person – and if it were possible, the person you'd have left would not be the same person you started with.[4]

And then there is the autistic artist Jon Adams, who said:

> Depression is like a coat you wear in summer. Whereas autism is who I am.[5]

I take this to mean that you can shed the coat and be more fully yourself. But if you shed the autism, there's no one left. I can relate to this because I also felt that my depression was taking me away from myself, rather than being an integral part of me. The absence of depression allowed me to be more, rather than less, authentic. This may be because I was lucky enough to recover fairly quickly. If I had been significantly debilitated over several years, perhaps I would have incorporated depression more fully into my sense of who I am.

I say this because there is some evidence that people who are disabled from birth feel very differently about their condition than do those disabled later in life (for example as a result of an accident).[6] For the first group, their sense of self seems to incorporate the ways in which they differ from others, and they can feel strong in who they are. Micheline Mason writes powerfully about this in her work *Incurably Human*.[7] In contrast, new or accidental disability is often accompanied with a genuine and understandable sense of loss and of diminution.

It is hard to be categorical about these issues, which are so abstract on the one hand, and variable between individuals on the other. Nonetheless, they have important implications in terms of attitudes towards, and classification of, the conditions in question. If depression is an illness, it has a rightful place in the diagnostic manuals for mental health professionals, the DSM or ICD. In contrast, if autism is a condition, a way of being, equally as fundamental as someone's sexuality,* or to the sum total of the perceptions of all their senses every second of every day, then does it belong in the list of mental health disorders?

The second thing that emerged from this sense that autism is fundamental to a person in the way that depression is not was a new set of questions about harm and suffering. Does autism

---

* Sexual orientation was rightly removed from the DSM in 1974 (although anxiety/ confusion over sexuality continued to be pathologised until 2013).

harm individuals? And if so, how? If autistic people suffer because the fluorescent lights are too bright, is the problem they experience akin to an illness that resides within their person, or do we need to change the lighting? If an autistic person suffers because they are being bullied for their difference, should we ask them to stop being autistic or tackle the malicious behaviour of the bullies? Should we treat autism with medication, or should we try to make the world a more autism-friendly place?

These questions led me to believe that autism did not cause Danny to suffer directly, and nor did his learning disability. The thing that brought about his agony, his tears, his screams, his aggression and self-injury was visceral bodily pain. When the pain was gone, he had a rather lovely life. He enjoyed listening to music, trampolining, swimming, funfairs, watching his favourite videos, using the swings and the climbing frames in the playground, being with his favourite people. He loved windy days and being driven along motorways. He loved sitting in his customary Buddha pose and tapping on shiny objects and the back of books or CD covers. If he needed medication, it was to reduce acid reflux, to promote intestinal motility, to take away pain and reduce spasm. What he didn't need was medication to stop him being himself. When talking about Danny's autism/learning disability, and when talking about gastrointestinal dysfunction, we were referring to completely different entities, only one of which, it seemed to me, warranted the label of being a disease.

I realise this is not the end of the matter. A lot has been written by others, and a lot more will go on being written. Even later in this book you might find me wobbling on these issues. I also know that 'selfhood' – or a sense of identity, or however you want to describe this sense we have of who we are – is a slippery and complicated thing that flows out into philosophy, psychology, neuroscience, sociology and politics (to name but a few of the potential academic fields).

Just over ten years later, with my depression now well-controlled on SSRIs, but still pondering the notion of identity and its relationship with autism, I would write in my journal:

What of Dan's identity? He has such a strong personality. And yet I have no idea how he constructs his sense of who he is (a sense I think he must have, because he gazes in the mirror a lot, and he smiles when I say how proud I am of him). I have so little clue as to what kind of narrative form his memories take (which they surely do, because he looks back at old photos, time and time again).

And when he is in pain he headbutts his reflection. Is this revealing? We have had to remove mirrors, and reflective surfaces, all over the house, because their predecessors all ended up as dangerous shards of glass or sharp plastic pieces on the floor.

Is this significant, at a cognitive or sensory or emotional level? I don't know.

I don't know much.

★

Here's another thing I don't know.

I don't know if it is fair to present the events of autumn 2003, incorporating the very darkest of hours for J and his family, as a catalyst for my own distress. Am I somehow leeching off their trauma, or expropriating it, in order to feed my own narrative?

What I can say is that the link between our families has endured and evolved since those dreadful days, thanks to J's family's magnanimity and the passage of time. J is now a happy and stable adult, supported to live in a community near to his parents, by an agency they trust. Even so, due to the parlous state of social care in the UK, and the vulnerability of adults such as J, his mother M ends an email to me with the phrase 'I will worry to the grave'.

Sometimes we dare to speak of the past.

M wants to know what I think happened back then. I speak of the lack of experience in the school at that time, TreeHouse trying to run before it could walk, that kind of thing. M endorses this interpretation and reminds me of the claims we made about TreeHouse – that we would become a centre of excellence – at a point when we were green and new and holding too much self-belief.

She says that J's gradual recovery at a residential school was thanks to the combined skills of an experienced and multidisciplinary staff team, and a more flexible approach.

So we go on to talk more broadly about ABA. We agree that ABA had been trumpeted as a great source of hope in the late 1990s, and that later such hope – in some people's cases at least – was rudely dashed. I venture to share accounts of those children for whom ABA had seemed beneficial, where it had provided a safe and enduring learning path to help the child build both self-esteem and trust in others. She says she has no doubt that it can be helpful for some, but also that it isn't appropriate for everyone. We can agree on this.

Then M's blue eyes fix me with a look of sadness for what has been, and of determination and belief for what might be.

'I do believe that everyone can be helped,' she says. 'It won't be the same thing for everyone. But everyone can be reached in some way. We just haven't found all the ways yet.'

Yes indeed. Let's not give up. Let's not give up on subgroups who don't fit with 'prototypical' autism, or those for whom schools can never be anything other than a source of torment. Let's not give up on people who don't respond to methods that most people recommend. Let's not give up on anyone.

There are so many ways to be human. There are so many ways to be autistic.

19

Debbie

After the desolate days of autumn 2003, I knew I was getting better when I attended the TreeHouse Christmas show. One of the pupils who had experienced a terrified meltdown the previous year was now, with evident pride and enjoyment, joining his classmates in a joke-telling stand-up routine. I reflected that we hadn't done right by J, but there were other pupils who were thriving, and there were other parents who were smiling and applauding. Perhaps the effort involved in helping TreeHouse on its way wasn't a damaging waste of energy after all.

Turning my gaze back into the world around me, I noticed some things that had passed me by for a while. PACE was struggling.

We had been fortunate in recruiting Armorer Wason to be director of PACE in 2001, but after she left to pursue international development work, we struggled to find a replacement. So I offered my services, free of charge, and was joined by a young star, Steve Broach. When he came to PACE he was prolific, bright, sensitive and supportive, with his own dose of mania too. Early on he told me that his real ambition was to become a barrister, so I knew we would be lucky if he stayed with us for long, but still, I thought, make the most of it. Working with Steve was terrific, and we remain friends to this day. I am proud to know him, and to see him feted by other disability campaigners as one of the leading human rights barristers of our time.[1]

★

The PACE office was used to taking calls from distressed parents. It was our role to give lobbying advice: write to your MP, go to their surgery, involve your local councillor, only engage the local press if you're absolutely sure it won't backfire, and so on. What we did not do, and never claimed to do, was individual casework. For this we would recommend a range of other more specialist advice and advocacy organisations.

Debbie was the exception. When she rang there was something so compelling about what she told me, and the way she told it, that I felt direct intervention was unavoidable.

What I learned from Debbie in that first phone call was as follows.

She was bright, witty, passionate, talkative. She was also autistic. Or I should say, given that the diagnostic criteria in those days distinguished Asperger syndrome from autism, she had been diagnosed with Asperger syndrome, as had both her sons.

Her attempts to secure educational provision that met the boys' needs had mutated into a child protection battle. She had been to tribunal twice. She had written endless letters, made multiple phone calls, and was seen as vexatious, troublesome, impossible to satisfy. Meanwhile, finding school increasingly intolerable, both her boys had started to refuse to attend.

'What can I do?' she said. 'They're big lads and I'm small. I can't physically force them to go to school. I'm not strong enough, for one thing.'

When she rang the PACE office, it was at a point when she thought her boys – Ben and Sam – were going to be taken away from her and her husband Michael, and instead placed in an institution or with foster parents.

She was deemed to be a bad mother, as if she was somehow manipulating them to dislike school, and now care proceedings had started. It was as if she was being punished for having the temerity to continue to make a case for her sons' educational needs. She was accused of using the children to meet her own emotional needs. Ben had myalgic encephalomyelitis (ME), also known as chronic fatigue syndrome, and this provided ammunition for professionals to question Debbie's mothering. Maybe he didn't really have ME at all; maybe instead this was a case of Fabricated or Induced Illness – or FII.

As touched on earlier, Fabricated or Induced Illness, a term that had replaced Munchausen Syndrome by Proxy, was an official category of child abuse concerning the invention or inducement of medical symptoms in a child by their caregiver (usually their mother). Increasingly, it seemed, parents of autistic children were under suspicion of inflicting this kind of abuse. This was partly because, as the writer, father and activist Mike Stanton pointed out, an official profile of a typical MSbP offender bore unfortunate resemblance to the characteristics you could easily find in many parents of autistic children. For example, such parents 'maintain a high degree of attentiveness' to their children; they 'typically shelter [them] from outside activities, such as school or play with other children' and so on. Stanton rightly reflected that this was actually what the autistic children often wanted and needed. He noted also that many who diagnosed MSbP knew very little about autism:

> Instead of attending to the child's needs they surmise that the parent is the one with problems and interpret all the evidence of need as proof of the parent's condition.[2]

This is not to downplay the seriousness of MSbP/FII when it truly occurs. But (and it's a big but) increasingly it seemed that MSbP/FII was being seized upon all too readily by professionals (and civil servants who wrote the guidance) whose reflex response to unusual children – or children who did not respond to orthodox treatments and approaches – was to suspect parents, rather than acknowledge their own helplessness in the face of invisible or incomprehensible distress in the children. It was even more likely that parents would be thus accused if their own communication styles were unusual, if they seemed in some way different. See where this leads? If you are a parent with so-called high-functioning autism, you may well arouse more suspicion in social, education and health professionals than do other, neurotypical parents – particularly if, like Debbie, you are unusually persistent when trying to make your point.

Debbie said that the GP had initially been supportive and had endorsed her concerns about Ben's chronic fatigue. But once social services began to assert that she was using her children as an attention-seeking device, the GP changed his tune. She had also sought the help of her local MP, who at first had been similarly supportive. But once social services started care proceedings, he too melted away.

Debbie felt as if all the systems that were supposed to protect them were instead hell-bent on undermining her and her family, closing in to break them apart.

In desperation, she lobbied even more energetically, trying to find someone who could help stop the juggernaut of child protection proceedings. She was amazingly good at this, if you take media coverage as a measure of effective campaigning. The Storeys' case was covered on *Channel 4 News*, Radio 4 and local media outlets.[3]

Unfortunately, though, the more people she contacted, the more it could be alleged that she was using her children as a way of getting attention for herself. And, perhaps, this made the professionals even more determined to dig in and persist in their chosen direction, rather than rewind and re-examine what had led to the rigidity of their stance.

I was oblivious to all of this until Debbie rang up the PACE office and said that someone at the Department for Education and Employment (DfEE) had suggested she try us. Whatever the route to us had been, here she was at the end of the phone asking for help. Because she had tried so many other sources of advice, support and assistance, and had already been such an effective campaigner, I was initially at a loss as to what more we could do. Yet there was something deeply compelling about Debbie, and about her situation.

The only thing for it, I felt, was to seek out the most eminent social worker in the country and see if he might help.

★

Herbert Laming's name was on all the guidance documents I dutifully read and summarised back in 1992, when I was employed at LSE to research community care. He was a big deal back then, as head of the Social Services Inspectorate.

Little did I know at the time that I would one day be introduced to him, via a strange series of links that would lead from Danny to TreeHouse to the House of Lords.

But now, in 2004, I was able to ring Tim Clement-Jones and ask him for Lord Laming's phone number. I briefly explained the problem to Tim, who understood immediately.

'Bastards,' he said.

Tim really does get the struggle of the underdog.

Luckily, Tim had already introduced me to Lord Laming, as a potentially helpful person in the TreeHouse story. Now I was to seek his help not specifically for TreeHouse but, instead, for a besieged family from Essex, whose problem was not autism per se but the way the system was victimising them rather than responding to their needs.

And what he did, once I had explained the situation, is quite simple – laughably simple, tragically, enragingly simple in a world where *who* you know is so very often more important than *what* you know. He gave me the name and number of the head of the children's services department in Debbie's local authority. He advised me to wait a day or two before contacting this person, during which time he would put in a good word and explain what to expect when I phoned.

The ensuing meeting with the director of the children's services department was surreal. Here were Steve and I telling this senior local authority officer and her professional colleagues about autism, and Asperger syndrome specifically. Steve had only recently graduated, and I was a mum who by chance found herself drawing the attention of high-ranking professionals to the seriousness of the knowledge gap in their department, and the resultant mistakes they had made.

We explained the social communication features of Asperger syndrome and hinted that the professionals may not have taken sufficient account of this in their relationship with Debbie. We also suggested, in the spirit of PACE's handbook *Constructive Campaigning*,[4] published the following year, that we were not seeking to blame individuals, but rather to address a wider system failure. The case highlighted the need for professionals to receive more training in autism and Asperger syndrome – conditions about which very little had been known until recently.

I am not sure if our visit had any long-term impact in that specific local authority. For Debbie, though, things started to change. She and the boys were allocated a new social worker and a new educational psychologist. There was a series of meetings with them, and they were calm and supportive. A new child protection meeting was convened, at which it was decided that the boys' names should be taken off the at-risk register and that care proceedings should cease. Debbie burst into tears, saying, 'This is so different from how the other meetings were', because the new chair was civil and respectful, rather than hostile and judgemental. I can only imagine how the previous meetings had been conducted. Debbie repeatedly thanked everyone, and repeatedly wept, and it seemed to me so sad that the system had made a pariah of this grateful, weeping, vulnerable, feisty, intelligent woman, who had simply fought passionately for her children.

So the boys were not taken away from Debbie and Michael, and over the Christmas of 2004, for the first time in an age, the family felt safe. Plans were made – in partnership rather than in conflict – for the gradual reintegration of Sam back into school. In contrast, it was agreed that it was no longer appropriate for Ben to return to a school he found hellish. Instead, approaching sixteen and therefore of an age when he had a legal right to make decisions about his own best interests, Ben chose home education, and his choice was upheld.

But there was no long-term rejoicing, because by the time we were into a new year, Debbie was desperately ill. She had been too frightened to go to the GP, who, she assumed, would once again believe she was merely attention-seeking. By the time she did receive medical attention, it was too late to arrest advanced and rapidly spreading cancer.

★

I went to visit Debbie in hospital on her last day. Her mother, Rosemarie, with huge emotional generosity, allowed me a few minutes with Debbie and Michael. I put some freesias on her pillow.

What was I expecting?

Not someone this ill, not *this* ill.

I had been a nurse and had seen people die, but still I was shocked. It was clear to me that I was intruding, clodhopping over a family's most precious intimate moments, but there I was in any case. As I sat with them, I longed to make Debbie a promise:

Debbie, I will make sure that your struggle remains in the public domain. I promise I will leave no stone unturned. I will make sure that things get better for other autistic children, parents, families, and this will be because of the inspiration your struggle has given me.

But it was too risky to say it; I should not promise something I might not be able to deliver. And certainly my capacity to deliver on anything was severely stretched soon after, and would be for many years. For example, I had to miss Debbie's funeral, because it clashed with a hospital appointment for Danny.

So instead, I told Debbie in those final minutes how glad I was to have known her, what a wonderful person she was, and what a great, great mother she was to her lovely sons.

20

REFLECTIONS

Years have passed, but the Storeys and I have stayed in touch.

It turned out there was a particular gene that would bring about not only Debbie's early death, but also that of her brother Neil and her sister Dee. Thus Jeff and Rosemarie would lose all three children to cancer, and the exhaustion and grief would perhaps be contributory factors in bringing on Rosemarie's dementia and Jeff's heart disease. But not before they heroically and doggedly continued to devote themselves to the survivors in their family, including Michael, Ben and Sam.

Jeff and Rosemarie worked hard throughout their adult lives, while bringing up three children. Jeff, as an engineer, would often work fifteen-hour days, and travel long distances either side of his working day. Rosemarie, as an operating theatre nurse, worked day and night shifts. They were law-abiding and they paid their taxes. When the system started to fail their family, they were initially stunned, and then angry.

When I first spoke to Jeff in 2004, about something to do with a statutory entitlement to an assessment, he said with a mix of exasperation and despair, 'You people ...'

And I knew that he was pointing out how hard the system is for so many, and that only some of us lucky ones manage to overcome the obduracy endemic in public institutions when they fail. His family had experienced education failures, social services failures, NHS failures, and had lost faith. In saying 'you people' he was referring to those of us for whom the system still works; 'we people' who still have the belief that if we talk the talk, backed up perhaps by posh accents and various qualifications, and know the right phrases to use and the right people, we will be OK. What the Storeys went through exemplified profound deficiencies in the institutions that are supposed to shield and protect us from adversity, but which instead failed a vulnerable family.

One of the more localised lessons I learned from those few months working alongside Debbie and her family was this:

We need to reform the social care workforce to respond better to the needs of disabled people and their families. Social workers who look at families only through the prism of potential abuse may actually inflict institutional abuse.

That's a bit dry. It would be hard to launch a battle cry or a soundbite on that. But it keeps me awake at night, as I still hear story after story of embattled, beleaguered families. Echoing this, I offer you an excerpt from my journal:

In an edition of *Special Needs Jungle*, there is a feature about how some social care professionals interpret parental requests for support as signs of parental failure:

'Parents being penalised or vilified for seeking support for their disabled child is not right in any society, yet it appears that in 21st century Britain this is perfectly acceptable in some LAs.' (Nathan Davies, Education Law Solicitor)

Aside from the deficiencies of the social care system, what else did I learn from Debbie and her family's story?

Above all, it highlighted for me once again the difference between autism and disease. And this fed a growing unease about the purpose, and potential pitfalls, of genomic research and treatment in relation to autism specifically, and learning disability more broadly.

Thinking of Debbie and her family, I could see unequivocally that I welcomed a possible future in which the cancer gene that ran riot through them might be eradicated from the gene pool. This might be through pre-implantation genetic testing (PGT),[1] or genome editing,[2] or some other yet-to-be-developed intervention method. So be it. Bring it on.

But I believed the same could absolutely *not* be said about any gene or genes that contributed to autism in the Storey family. Rosemarie once said she thought she probably had Asperger's, like two of her three children and her grandsons. But, actually, so what? It conferred considerable skills and personality attributes on them all, even while in some areas it held them back. Until cancer struck, they thrived. They were a big, united family, quirky, for sure, with some challenges, for sure – but then, who doesn't have quirks and challenges? It was not their autism that cut down three siblings in their prime, robbed parents of their children and children of their parents.

This is why, when some people used to complain about disparities between expenditure on cancer research and autism research, or the superior availability of cancer treatment in contrast with autism treatment, others of us were shocked at the very idea that this is a relevant comparison.[3]

And this is also why, when I hear that whole genome sequencing is to go ahead, with a view, possibly, to eliminating 'serious' or 'severe' conditions, I feel a chill. How very, *very* careful we have to be, in deciding what we mean by 'serious', or what counts as 'severe'. It seems deceptively straightforward if a decision not to have a child is based on a prognosis of an extremely short life that will consist of unremitting pain. (Bioethicists usually cite Tay-Sachs as the definitive condition in this category.[4]) But where do we draw the line? At what point does some potential condition's propensity to cause suffering become too trivial to justify a concerted effort to prevent it? Susceptibility to certain non-fatal cancers? Potential osteoporosis? Acne? Dyslexia? Most lives offer a quantity and quality of experience that is preferable to no life at all – something that is acknowledged even among ethicists who tend to be enthusiastic about preventing disability.[5]

And who are the 'we' who make the decisions – the people who live out these conditions or the onlookers who pass judgement? We know, from the example of MSbP/FII in Debbie's case, that outsiders can often get it wrong, and we also know that ideas about which kinds of life are worthwhile – and which are not – can evolve and change. The more people I would meet who earned a diagnosis of autism, the more frequently I would reject the tendency of neurotypicals to pathologise it.

Part 4

THE WHIRLWIND YEARS, 2006–9

'If everybody looked the same
We'd get tired looking at each other.'

Groove Armada, 'If Everybody
Looked the Same'

In the ten years following Danny's diagnosis in 1996, my circumstances had changed dramatically. I had gone from being an isolated mother at home to a campaigner who sometimes found herself on TV and radio, in conferences and parliamentary meetings. Thanks to Danny I had found new friends, including autism academics and other parents – people I might otherwise never have met.

But 2006 ushered in yet more changes. During the next three years I would set out on a course of study that would eventually lead to a doctorate, I would have life-changing encounters with leading figures in the neurodiversity movement, and I would meet the Queen and Arsène Wenger, not to mention my future husband and stepsons.

Where was I in the middle of it all? I was Danny's mum. Of this central identity I could be sure, and my chief preoccupation was trying to get treatment for his escalating health problems. What I could be much less sure of was where I fitted in the wider autism community; battles seemed to be raging all around, as if I was in some kind of war zone. What was my natural milieu? What circle did I move in, and which echo chamber did I occupy?

21

JOHN

September 2006

I thought a ride in a pod on the London Eye would be an exciting birthday treat for Danny as he entered his teenage years, and it would also offer a relaxed and informal setting for John – a new potential carer – to meet all sides of the extended family.

I still have the photo taken on the descent. Here at the front is Danny, sitting on the floor of the pod, in his customary legs-crossed pose, elbows on knees, cupping his face in his hands. Here too are Ingrid, Jack and Ben; Nick with Amanda and their little boys Lowell and Jesse; Paul and Daniel Collier; Hornby cousins; TreeHouse friends; and me. Right at the back, his forehead just discernible behind Ingrid's irrepressible hair, is John.

Given the potential dangers – all the usual things that babies and toddlers can do, not to mention the unpredictable responses of the young autistic passengers, to the height, the confinement and the close proximity to people they haven't met before – why did I think this would be fun for any of us? I wonder now how we pulled off an organised photo, all nineteen passengers clustered together as required and facing the camera just in time for the flash. Indeed, how did we all manage to get on to a moving platform in the first place? And then stay cheerful and positive throughout the ride, and finally pile off in time for the next passengers to board?

All of this was ambitious enough. But what I didn't know is that John *hates* heights. For John, a ride on the London Eye was the worst kind of introduction imaginable. Yet instead of feigning sickness or another commitment, he turned up that Saturday morning, smiled and chatted his way through the ride, and passed with flying colours.

Maybe he said to himself, 'If I can cope with this, I can cope with anything' – which is pretty much what John has had to do throughout the ensuing seventeen years. He has been with Danny and his extended family at times of confusion, distress, anxiety and celebration. When we first met him he was a student nurse, who came to us via a colleague of Sarah's. In time he would become a senior nurse at Great Ormond Street Hospital. He has met challenge after challenge, excelling always.

He has instigated regular trips to the Highbury Barn pub, so that Danny can hang out cheerfully with Nick and family and become a welcome and familiar customer in his local. If you heard the jokes, the insults and football banter during these pub visits, you'd recognise in John a hardcore Scouser, the finest that Liverpool has to offer. He is a lifelong Everton supporter, and capable of all the turmoil that goes with such an allegiance. But don't be fooled by the stereotype. The deep and abiding love and loyalty he gives to everyone who needs him are plain to see. And heaven knows, Danny – and the rest of us – have so often needed him.

22

Larry, and the Wider Autism Movement

By the time of John's arrival in our lives, TreeHouse and PACE were in the process of merging, and had jointly moved to yet another temporary building – this one, at last, on our newly acquired Muswell Hill site.

It was a relief to be able to expand the school once again and for the first time not dread the prospect of the inevitable next move. We could also expand our wider work. With even greater personal relief, I was able to hand over the national development role that I had held on a voluntary basis, to a highly regarded professional within the field of SEN – Linda Redford. I found in her a great colleague, with her humour, kindness and integrity. Her arrival allowed me to contemplate a reduction in work hours and a gradual departure from the charities that had, with Danny, been my life. I could sense that it might – just – be possible to return to some kind of academic work, and also gain some experience beyond TreeHouse/PACE into the wider world of autism.

I stood as a candidate for the National Autistic Society's council, and from there I would become a trustee for four years. I joined at an interesting time. A seismic shift in the orientation of the NAS was taking place. The 'nothing about us without us' demands of the disability rights movement could no longer be ignored. The social model of disability was no longer seen merely as a sidelines perspective; the voices of autistic 'self-advocates' were now recognised as relevant and compelling. Chief among the movers who were effecting this change was Larry Arnold.

★

'Just because someone has a diagnosis of autism, it doesn't mean they're going to be a good board member.'

This was what I first heard about Larry. He had recently been elected onto the NAS board of trustees – the first autistic person to join. Until then it had been dominated by parents.

I had not yet met Larry, but I was curious about my colleague's scepticism.

'Basically, Larry isn't a very nice person,' I was told.

I did not think to ask if niceness had been on the trustee person spec. Instead I asked for further explanation.

'He's really aggressive and he frightens people.'

'Oh? In what way?'

It seemed that some of this assessment was attributable to his wearing a hat, and walking with a stick, and having lots of facial hair, and being prone to talking loudly.

I could imagine it would be hard to ignore such a person, but was puzzled by the implication that such characteristics disqualified him from trusteeship.

Then the killer judgement, which I have heard often, from other neurotypicals, in different places at different times: 'Just because someone's autistic, it doesn't mean they should get away with being rude.'

Think about this one. Certain aspects of perceived rudeness, we all surely know, are down to culture. Some cultures say 'please' and 'thank you' more than others; some value eye contact more than others; some have differences in intonation and rhythm that may make their sentences sound abrupt or staccato compared with other cultures, when actually the people talking are feeling perfectly relaxed and friendly. And think of the subtle errors in translation that can happen when people speak in different languages.

For example, how often have we heard a gifted linguist from another country affirm something in English by saying 'of course'? They don't mean 'you're stating the obvious, you idiot', but it can come over like that. And then again there are just personality differences: one person's well-meaning curiosity might be another person's intrusiveness; one person's diplomacy might be another person's sycophancy. It is important to recognise the difference between intended and unintended rudeness, and to hold back on too readily taking offence.

So, if my colleague who did not like Larry was right – that he seemed frightening and angry and rude – was this because he had fewer boot-licking skills than many of us, due to his autism, or just that he may have had to fight harder than others to get to where he was, given that by definition his social communication style may have been alien to others? And had it occurred to her that the issue of class might have seeped into her opinion? As well as being autistic, Larry has a strong West Midlands accent, and he is emphatically working class. At a time when many candidates for trusteeship were eligible by virtue of their connections and their professions, did this additional component of Larry's difference play into her doubt about him?

*

I had the opportunity to meet Larry for myself at my first meeting of the NAS council.

He was having a bad day. A really, really bad day. He was interrupting people, he was agitated, he spoke louder and louder, over the top of them, and there were several impassioned outbursts from him, which drew strong reproaches from others.

'Shh, Larry!'

'Larry, be quiet!'

'*Larry!*'

He subsided eventually.

And then, a few days later, I read a mortified, deeply apologetic email from him, sent to the whole council email group. I have known many NTs who seem incapable of ever apologising, or re-examining past behaviour. But because of this email, I learned very quickly that Larry reflects on things a lot, and is prone to be very hard on himself.

For the next few years, the NAS council email group proved to be a source of fascination: a mix of opinions and factual updates, in which some members were prolific and others silent. Larry's contributions stood out for the breadth of his intellectual range, his passion and his depth of knowledge. We did not always agree, but he always made me think.

It was from Larry I learnt the term 'curebie', which referred to the collective of parents and scientists who sought a cure for autism, and who also were likely to believe that the MMR vaccine had brought it about, and/or that biomedical treatments should be investigated and tried, even if they were unlicensed and backed with limited evidence. The curebie culture presented autism as so awful that it was worth trying extreme measures to deal with it. Chelation was one such example, as was extensive hormone treatment.[1]

I was with Larry, but only up to a point.

Despite the horrendous lengths to which some rogue practitioners would go, I could understand those parents who wanted a cure for autism – *if* they believed it was inextricably linked with physical illness, such as gastrointestinal problems. If I had thought autism was to blame for Danny's GI problems, I might have become as desperate. So I was enthusiastic about responsible research into, and cure of, the GI problems that Danny had, and I was concerned when scientists and autistic advocates alike just dismissed them as irrelevant.*

I remember one of Larry's emails in which he said he was fed up with hearing from parents about their autistic children screaming in pain. I found this troubling in its bluntness, though I recognised his broader point – there are many painful conditions that blight our lives, regardless of our neurotype, and GI problems are found across the population.

In any case, he was not the only person to be blunt. When I joined him on the trustee board, I was amazed to witness a fellow trustee (NT) shouting at him, 'Shut *up*, Larry, *shut up!*' And what's more, this person was later congratulated by a fellow (NT) trustee for doing so.

It seemed to me then, as now, that we were experiencing one rule for NTs and another for autistics. In this company, if NTs were rude, it was because they had been provoked by an autistic person. But if autistics were rude, it was because they were autistic. Either way, autistic people got the blame. This was profoundly dissonant for a charity that claimed to champion the rights of autistic people, and which called on outsiders to understand – and make reasonable adjustments for – the very condition that some of the trustees themselves seemed to dislike so much.

---

* For a while I became involved in a charity –Visceral – that supposedly raised money for broad research into GI problems among autistic people. It soon became clear to me, however, that its real purpose was much more limited. Namely, it was to support Wakefield's quest to prove himself right – and to pay him rather generously in the process. I resigned, though I avoided the tough conversations I perhaps should have had.

At a subsequent council meeting, held in an unfamiliar hotel venue, I heard a small commotion, a familiar raised voice near the reception area. Larry was speaking loudly and agitatedly. I went to see if I could help, and for a while was just there on standby to mediate if necessary. It got sorted – an issue about his room – and Larry managed to calm himself. And here's the thing I realised about Larry: a lot of the time, Larry is really anxious. I could see how quickly he was breathing, I could almost hear the rapidity of his heart rate, and sense the fight-or-flight chemicals coursing through his body. There was no ill will behind Larry's raised voice. His agitation was linked to his feeling of vulnerability.

And from then on I knew not to find him disconcerting, and this enabled me to discover so many wonderful things about the treasure trove that is Larry. He would make us all laugh with his wit later that day in the council meeting, and he would say things that required us to think about our own standpoints. I learned how hard it is for him to travel between Coventry and London so frequently for endless meetings, because of the sensory overload, the anxiety around unexpected change, the sheer determination required to overcome all the unpleasantness entailed.

'So what keeps you involved in all this campaigning?' I asked Larry over lunch at my last council meeting. 'Does it get any easier?'

'It's like walking on glass,' he replied. 'It goes on hurting as much, but you just get used to it.'

So I came to know that Larry is a kind, brave, funny man with a towering intellect, a man of many talents and interests. He played the flute, he went to Wales every Christmas because he loved the landscape and would share his beautiful photographs online, he was a passionate cultivator of his allotment, and he – like me – was embarking on a doctorate. Later, he would single-handedly establish and edit the online journal

Autonomy (to which I would be a one-off, minor contributor) and we would share a speaking slot at a conference. So you will meet Larry again later in the story, but for now I want to share one more recollection.

★

I am driving Larry and our mutual friend Dinah back to her house one morning after the three of us have met for coffee.

He is in the passenger seat and he is talking while I drive. He speaks with authority about the architectural features of the buildings we pass; he notices details about my locality that I've failed to see for three decades.

I am about to pull away as the traffic light turns from red and amber to green and suddenly a cyclist shoots across us from the right. I break sharply, just narrowly missing him, and both Dinah and I emit sounds of shock and indignation.

'Sorry,' says Larry. 'Was I talking too much and distracting you?'

While the cyclist sped off, unharmed and no doubt oblivious, here was Larry blaming himself for something of which he was entirely innocent.

I give this story to you as an important example of Larry's capacity for self-doubt, and his ability to offer apology. I think it may surprise many of the people who, in the past, have judged Larry, as some of those early NAS colleagues did, based on an incomplete first impression. While inflexibility is supposedly a feature of autism, it was no less apparent in the attitudes of Larry's neurotypical critics.

23

TRIBALISM

In the autumn of 2007, a 'bitter ideological war' was the focus of extensive media attention in the UK.[1] A series of letters in the *Independent* newspaper,[2] and a debate on the influential BBC Radio 4 *Today* programme,[3] addressed a new campaign by the National Autistic Society.

This was the Think Differently About Autism campaign,[4] which aimed to raise awareness of autism, presenting it not as a disease or as something to be feared and lamented, but rather as a different way of being, to be accepted and even welcomed as part of natural human diversity.

Not everyone supported this shift of emphasis, this move away from the overwhelmingly negative or sensationalist ways autism had usually been portrayed in the past. Critics of the campaign, as exemplified by some of the *Independent* letter writers, felt strongly that it was a misleading and inaccurate whitewash of the difficulties that autistic people experience. Instead, they argued that there was an urgent need to find treatments, therapies and causes for a condition that – some felt – might ideally not exist at all.

The debate aroused passions on both sides of the argument. For some autistic people and those close to them, the time to

recognise them as individuals with strengths and positive qualities was long overdue. Yet for others – often family members of
autistic people who were severely disabled – it felt that merely
to 'accept' autism, without intervening to help affected individuals overcome some of their difficulties, was tantamount to
negligence and neglect.

There seemed to be a binary divide about who is best placed
to advocate for autistic people and to judge on the relative merits
of contrasting interventions. On the one hand there were able
autistics who challenged the overwhelmingly negative ways in
which autism was portrayed – usually by neurotypical academics
and parents. They questioned an exclusive emphasis on impairments and failure to recognise autistic strengths, asserted autism
as an identity and criticised the paternalism that had dominated
their treatment until now. On the other hand, external experts
and many parents often pointed to the difficulties that autistic
people experienced, and the additional challenges for those who
could not use words, and/or with severe learning disabilities
and/or distressed and violent behaviours.

I could see and respect both points of view. Getting to know
autistic adults like Debbie and Larry – likable, funny, admirable
and kind – convinced me that an emphasis solely on the impairments was not only unfair but also inaccurate. I knew this in a
different way about Danny, whose capacity for pleasure and
contentment had contagious qualities. Still, I felt that the notion
of 'self-advocacy' was inapplicable for someone like Danny,
whose frame of reference was so very limited, due to his difficulties in comprehension and communication. He would always
need me, and others, to advocate on his behalf. Also, I was
aware that even some able and articulate autistics disputed the
'acceptance' position.

Whose voice do we listen to? How do we square it if some
people like and assert their differences, while others wish only
to be 'normal'?

This debate also required me to address once again the perennial question of how autism should be conceptualised. How to unify in a coherent way the disparate abilities and qualities of Danny and many of his fellow pupils at TreeHouse, with those of the so-called high-functioning autistic people I met? What, truly, did they have in common sufficient to justify a shared diagnosis? I was familiar with Simon Baron-Cohen's position regarding 'the extreme male brain', whereby male brains were considered to be strong in 'systemising' (as opposed to empathising) and autistic brains were explained as an extreme version of this.[5] But I couldn't relate this to all of the autistic people I knew. The idea that autistic people might be particularly good at understanding and building systems such as computers and machinery, as well as abstract concepts in the arts or politics, was all very well, but if I was to explain *Danny's* autism to a newcomer with reference to the extreme male brain, it was baffling at best, insufficient for sure, and – if I'm honest – it felt irrelevant to gaining a better understanding of what made him tick.

Of greater significance, had I known of it at the time, would have been an article about 'monotropism' that had been published in 2005.[6] This would only come my way years later, by which time I had formed a friendship with its principal author, Dinah Murray.

The article proposed that autistic people's facility for intense focus and interests (*monotropism*) differed crucially from the more diffuse attention and interest systems (*polytropism*) in neurotypicals. This difference, it argued, was at the root of the behavioural differences described in the triad of impairments, and could explain the whole range of abilities across the spectrum, for example, propensities for both linguistic ability among the so-called high-functioning, and inability to acquire speech at all among the non-verbal. In addition, it explained the strength of emotions – the intensity, the passions – that accompanied autistic enthusiasms on the one hand, or meltdowns on the other: 'individuals on the autism spectrum tend to be either passionately interested or not interested at all'.[7]

This interpretation gave greater credence to the subjective experiences of autistic people than had other theories. It was notable that the article's authors were themselves autistic.

Even though I was not aware of this article at the time, I was keen to learn from the able autistic people I met about how they perceived the world. After all, it was autistic adults with the power to speak and write who had helped to shift mainstream thinkers towards recognising the significance of sensory differences in autism. The people I met were not just incredibly interesting in themselves, they also helped me to understand Danny better, and see that a behaviour that outsiders might consider to be 'meaningless' or 'mindlessly repetitive' or 'infantile' could have significance and value.

You will hear more about Dinah Murray later in our story. More will also emerge about developments in scientific exploration that seek to build on the testimony, knowledge and experience of autistic people.[8] But the relevance of all of this for me during the early 2000s lay in the growing sense of a chasm opening up, between different wings of the autism community.

It seemed that for many, it was not enough simply to accept that the autism spectrum embraced an enormous range of personalities and abilities and that many different voices (including parental and sibling voices) could coexist. Rather, it seemed that some wanted to compete for authenticity and legitimacy, and disregard the experiences of others, claiming to be the sole voice, or to have the most valid perspective on life as an autistic person. This contrast would later be referred to as a dispute about 'brand ownership'.[9]

I felt that this divide was too binary for the realities of life on the spectrum. For one thing, it disregarded all those in 'the big middle',* whose abilities and difficulties didn't fit in an arbitrary division. For another thing, it disguised the extent to which an autistic person might be very able in one area and yet struggle significantly in others. The hard-hitting film made by Amanda Baggs brought this truth home forcefully. It demonstrated how some autistic people can be highly intelligent and eloquent, while never acquiring the ability (or desire) to speak, and while always needing extensive support in personal care and other aspects of daily life.[10] The sentiments have been echoed in the important phrase, 'Just because I don't speak doesn't mean I have nothing to say.'[11] However, others felt that Amanda Baggs's film did a disservice to the non-verbal autistics who would never acquire her intellectual grasp or her ability to deploy extensive vocabularies or complex ideas.

This area is fraught with potential dangers of overgeneralisation. While Amanda Baggs opened up the important possibility that apparently non-verbal people may have a powerful intellect, there was a risk that this potential would be presumed to be universal when it was not. In the case of Danny, I never wanted to underestimate his capacity for learning, or the validity of his inner thoughts and ideas, however inaccessible some of them might be to me. On the other hand, I felt it was supremely important not to project onto him a fantasy of who he might be, and in so doing undervalue the person he was and is. To fixate on the possibility or hope that he might read and type one day felt like a denial of his integral value as he was in the absence of these skills. To my mind, a man who still prefers to watch childhood videos of Fireman Sam in his late twenties, and who is disinclined to seek out activities that contain academic potential of any kind, is no lesser a person than a man who races through quantum physics texts with ease.

---

* Thanks to Adrian Whyatt for introducing me to this phrase.

Another phenomenon I observed was the tendency of some parents (those of the most learning-disabled autistics) to envy the more able – the 'Asperger type' autistics. In so doing, they assumed that the more intellectually able had an easier ride. I question this. They may need less support in their daily lives, but some of the so-called 'mildly' autistic people experience some of the worst ravages of self-loathing and rage, the most dramatic and violent meltdowns of all, the greatest sense of despair and isolation, feeling and fearing that they may never 'belong', that they may never find their tribe.

It's not a competition for suffering, nor for achievement, despite some people's attempts to present it as such. Even so, for as long as this tension about autism's essence exists, it is accompanied by a tension about whether, why and in what way autism requires 'intervention'. And this brings me back to the earlier discussion about ABA, which, as I said, threads itself in and out of Danny's and my story like a snake.

I now want to introduce you to someone who has challenged me to the core in this regard.

24

ABA Tribes and Michelle Dawson

At a time when I was learning from Larry and others about the neurodiversity movement, I ran slap-bang into an article about ABA that sent me into a tailspin. This was an essay by Michelle Dawson: 'The Misbehaviour of Behaviourists'.[1]

Until then I had heard only vaguely about Michelle as the autistic woman who had submitted a legal challenge against a Supreme Court of Canada judgment that ABA for autistic children was medically necessary.[2] 'The Misbehaviour of Behaviourists' referred to the poor quality of contrasting research studies into autism. I was at that point unaware of how qualified she was to make such judgements. I did not know of her impressive credentials as a research scientist working with Professor Laurent Mottron in Montreal, nor of her wide reputation for forensic analysis of a vast array of the autism literature – something that later earned her an honorary doctorate.

So when I came to read the article, I knew only that she was fiercely critical of many of the practices and claims made by proponents of ABA. In the UK, I had found that opposition to ABA was often expressed in ways that revealed outdated preconceptions and limited knowledge of how practitioners really worked. As such, I had not taken the criticisms very seriously.

But suddenly I was hearing new arguments from Michelle. I now read that ABA practitioners were not, after all, viewed as people who believed in the potential of autistic children and who refused to write them off as 'unteachable'. Rather, it seemed they were taskmasters who were trying to stop autistic people being autistic. I read that ABA was not the intervention of hope and belief, of evidence-based practice and impeccable commitment to research; instead, it was the intervention of oppression, bad science, charlatans and commercial interests. And I learned that 'advocates' – chiefly parent campaigners such as me and many of my colleagues – were often dangerous and wrong-headed. And that we were oblivious to the issue of rights – the right to be autistic, the right not to be patronised, the right of autistic people themselves to figure out what their needs were, rather than having parents or professionals decide them on autistic people's behalf.

Fuck. Had I been doing the work of the devil all this time? Had I inadvertently been causing major offence to the very community of people I thought I had been helping?

I showed Michelle Dawson's article to a behaviour analyst colleague, and my heart sank when all this person could say was: 'Well it's a rant, isn't it?'

Full stop.

'But what do you think of the points she's making, about human rights, and the way autistic people are being devalued, and her challenge to the rigour of the ABA outcome studies?'

'It's a rant, it's not an academic article.'

This refusal to engage in a conversation, or to self-question, was deeply dispiriting. It was as if anything other than a peer-reviewed article with graphs and p-values and esoteric behavioural terminology was of no interest, and that any alternative form of enquiry or intellectual position was irrelevant or inferior. And it was a refusal to address the all-important question of why or how the same intervention can be perceived by some as helpful, and by others as harmful. Most of the ABA practitioners I met were fuelled by kindness and a fondness for and interest in the children; they were bright, talented, motivated, brave and patient. Yet I couldn't help noticing that there were a handful – particularly at an academic level – who seemed remote, distanced and unaware of how to build a rapport with the children they were employed to help; who were arrogant and dismissive of the knowledge possessed by other professionals, neurodivergent people and parents, and disinclined to enter into discussion with dissenters.[3]

Despite this, I continued to participate in an echo chamber in which ABA was endorsed and welcomed. I read post after enthusiastic post on a UK-wide email group – parental accounts in which positive, hopeful and in some cases transformative applications of ABA were helping children to learn, find pleasure and resort less frequently to desperate and harmful outbursts brought about by intense emotion or communication failures. It was taken as gospel that ABA had the best claim to evidence to support its impact. And until reading 'The Misbehaviour of Behaviourists', the arguments I had heard against ABA were chiefly based on rumours originating from the early repellent uses of ABA, practices that, I had thought, were long gone.

But the article opened a Pandora's box. It required me to think again, and to take some tentative steps into new arenas, to venture into new echo chambers in which very different experiences of ABA were discussed.

'The Misbehaviour of Behaviourists' led me to seek out Michelle in person, first via email and eventually face to face. Fortunately, she visited the UK in 2012 to give a series of presentations including a keynote speech at the NAS Professional Conference.[4]

Email conversations with Michelle had shown her to be friendly and open as well as clever, but it was only when I met her that I found also humour, and a kind of sadness too – a disarming combination of strength and vulnerability and warmth. I would struggle to remember any of the contents of our discussion, so overwhelmed was I by the non-verbal messages and the emotional power of meeting her. I would continue to be outclassed intellectually by her subsequent correspondence with me.

Suffice it to say that, as I look back at my meeting with Michelle, and the conversations I have had with advocates from the neurodiversity movement over the years, it feels as if I have been trying to balance on a broken seesaw ever since. On one end sit the ABA-lovers, and on the other end sit the ABA-haters. It too often feels as if all participants are hell-bent on driving the seesaw up and down as vigorously as they can, seeking to unseat their opponent at the top of their rise, and preparing for the next killer thrust as they descend.

And here I stand, wobbling, one foot on either side of the central pivot, trying to hold my balance as the weight of different opposing arguments threatens to toss me into the air or plunge me to the ground. I want to stop this back-and-forth competition, in which both sides are fuelled by simultaneous feelings of righteousness and victimhood.

The parallel echo chambers fail to agree even about what ABA really is. It becomes a struggle of meaning and knowledge, depending on whose side you're on. For those who believe in the benefits of ABA, any examples of harm are dismissed as bad practice, or not real ABA. In contrast, for those who are convinced of the badness of ABA, any illustrations that seem beneficial are, by definition, 'not really ABA at all'.

This tribal animosity is vicious, particularly on social media. It means that only the most zealous – or the most brave – are willing to put their heads above the parapet. Opinions harden, people stop listening to one another, or they believe they know what others are going to say before they've even said it. The neurodiversity movement's standpoint becomes dismissed by many people in the ABA hierarchy, while pro–ABA advocates are subjected to 'no platforming' policies by some autistic self-advocates and their allies. It's grim.

But it's not just a struggle of meaning and knowledge, a quest for truth. For me it is also a struggle of the heart, and a struggle of what feels like competing solidarities. It feels as if I somehow have to choose between, on the one hand, so many parents, TreeHouse, Danny himself who enjoyed his ABA so much, and, on the other hand, those critics of ABA with whom I have come to agree on other issues, to recognise and respect their powerful intellects, and to like and admire enormously. I want instead to ask them all to come to rest, converse, stop taking up opposing and extreme positions, engage with one another, listen and learn. I want to say (as I did in a conference speech in Galway[5]) words to the effect of:

Let's stop trying to score points off one another, and let's try and avoid a 'heroes and villains' mentality. This is not a game of football. We're not talking about unconditional team loyalty in which, in order to love your side, you have to hate the opponents. It's not a fight to see who wins and who loses, who gets a red card and who scores.

I believe we have to pause here and reflect on how this polar-isation came about, and what factors poured fuel on the flames. Here are some thoughts about how the conflict is understood, how it has been communicated, and where I hope we may get to.

I have recently read concerning reports about how some USA-based ABA providers are driven by the commercial prior-ities of private equity companies.[6]

And this reminded me of an idea I had several years back, about the impact of the funding and cultural context in which autism interventions are delivered. Michelle Dawson's challenge to the idea that ABA is 'medically necessary' for autistic children always seemed valid to me. I do wonder how many parents deep down believed that ABA was *medically* necessary – or did they just feel compelled to present their cause in such terms in order to get help for their children?

Let's explore the context. First of all, the growth of ABA for autistic children happened at a time when very little of any kind of help was available. So when the Lovaas research came out, it was seized upon as a source of help and hope. But families needed to access funding to run a home programme. Given the medical diagnostic category of autism, and in places where private medical insurance was the norm, perhaps it was expedient to present autism as a medical problem, and one sufficiently urgent to justify prolonged 'treatment' leading to 'recovery'.

In addition, actuarial calculations on which private medical insurance is based presumably looked to the possibility that early intervention could save money long term. So an intervention through which autistic children can 'recover' made good commercial sense for the insurers, particularly if they were convinced by the research. The 'gold standard' type of intervention research is the randomised controlled trial (RCT) – and Lovaas and colleagues had managed to conduct something approaching this.

Critics – Dawson included – would later highlight the inadequacies of the Lovaas research. They would also question the reliability and independence of subsequent studies, particularly where the researchers were the same people who stood to gain financially or reputationally. It was for this reason that some held the ABA industry to be part of a 'medical-industrial complex'.*

In the UK, though, the financial and institutional climate is altogether different. Here, the language and goals linked to early

---

* Dinah used this term in a conversation with me.

intervention have tended to emphasise educational need rather than medical prognosis. As such, goals are set in terms of educational progress rather than recovery. This perhaps reflects a cultural contrast, but – more significantly I believe – less reliance is placed on crude actuarial calculations in the UK because the cost of future care will come from a different organisation's budget. Instead of making a case to private medical insurance companies, parents in the UK have looked to public sector funding and specifically SEN and disability law, and the requirements of the prevailing inspectorates (Ofsted and the Care Quality Commission (CQC), for example).

This has a significant impact on the language around autism and ABA, and it also means that evidence of efficacy at an SEN tribunal relies not on the RCT-type study, but on demonstrations of progress for an individual in relation to their unique, personal goals. This in turn permits a far more nuanced approach, where practitioners can be guided by behavioural science to devise and measure *specific interventions relevant to each child* – improvements in ability to communicate perhaps, use of signs, new strategies for coping with public transport, or learning to take crucial medication. In other words, it means that the practice need not be governed by the need to comply with the requirements of a randomised trial, but can be tailored to each unique child's motivations and environment. Meticulous data is taken to evaluate progress against specific areas of learning, rather than to conform to a uniform set of standardised scales of autism symptoms.

This does not take the heat completely out of the argument, but it does lower the temperature. It perhaps explains why the work and goals of so many UK-based practitioners would be unrecognisable to the original Lovaas therapists. It explains too why many UK-based behaviour analysts are as appalled at the misuse of their science – to quell stims for example, to promote 'camouflaging' – as are their critics in the neurodiversity movement.[7]

I have recently been talking with Esther, one of Danny's current support team. Esther is passionate about her work with autistic children and adults. She says working with Danny is like going to see a friend. She trained as a teacher in Spain – the country of her birth – and worked with children with special needs. She then came to the UK to pursue her interest in ABA. She has studied and trained and practised for several years, and is a qualified Board Certified Behaviour Analyst (BCBA).

To the sceptics and enemies of ABA, she is thereby damned.

But listen to this:

Esther stood up at a conference in Europe to challenge a particularly rigid old-school-ABA speaker, who was suggesting that therapists should be aiming for 'normal' and 'age-appropriate' behaviour. Esther was and is appalled that a learning-disabled adult (like Danny) should be stopped from watching kiddies' cartoons or playing with his soft toys in case he is stigmatised by wider society. Esther knows that actually most people who meet Danny are not judgemental at all, because they can quickly see that he is learning disabled. Rather, they are charmed by his manifest pleasure in his chosen pursuits, can appreciate the rationale for allowing him access to the things that bring him such evident and contagious joy. Likewise we are both appalled that – in the view of some so-called experts – it is apparently OK for neurotypical twenty-five-year-olds to participate in video games such as *Grand Theft Auto* (in which the player can have sex with a prostitute and then get their money back by killing her)* but not OK to enable an adult of the same age to visit a children's playground and go on a swing, even if they derive huge enjoyment from it.

Esther uses her skills and her love to help guide the people she supports. She knows to be completely flexible according to

---

* *Grand Theft Auto* (GTA) is a videogame series that has achieved global popularity, with sales in the hundreds of millions.

their interests and how they're feeling on any particular day. And in her rejection of so much of the previous normalising orthodoxy, she is by no means alone in the evolving and developing field of ABA in the UK.*,**

So there is a battle of ideas within the ABA movement as well. I believe there is scope for reform, and that one day notions of recovery and normalisation will fade away from the discourse. Instead, skilled practitioners can get on with the job of teaching and guiding according to the needs of each person.

If you make it to the end of this book, you may find there are signs of hope.

---

* The UK Society for Behaviour Analysis has now set up a register and is also developing its own supervision and competence standards for behaviour analytic professionals, which might contribute to further distancing from the harshest and least helpful applications of behaviour analysis.

** An interesting and contemporary account of how ABA practice has been used on behalf of four very different autistic boys is offered by Sarah Ziegel in her 2022 book, *Marching to a Different Beat: A family's journey with autism.*

25

ARSENAL AND ARSÈNE WENGER

Who would have thought that, thanks to Danny, I would get to meet some of the legendary characters of the Premier League? But so it came to pass: Arsenal and TreeHouse came together in a productive union for one glorious football season.

The news that TreeHouse had been chosen as Arsenal's charity of the season (2007–8) came through to me on my mobile phone, just as I was walking away from an event in parliament. Unable to contain my joy, I kind of danced and screamed right there on the pavement of Parliament Street, as if I had just won the EuroMillions, or *The X Factor:* something totally stupendous and once-in-a-lifetime had happened.

Oh. My. God. Oh my GAAAD.

★

'You do realise,' Linda said to some of my colleagues, 'that Virginia may, literally, explode, when Arsène and the players visit.'

She was referring to the first visit to TreeHouse that Arsène Wenger (feted manager of Arsenal Football Club) and Gael Clichy and Gilberto Silva (two of his star players) were about to make.

This was unquestionably the most exciting day of my life. A day that still, in retrospect, compensates for all the heartache and anxiety and exhaustion that went into the TreeHouse years and beyond. It was also one of the most profoundly rewarding outcomes of my marriage to Nick (who, unfortunately for him, was out of the country on the day of the visit). Divorce had in no way damaged our joint endeavour with Danny, nor had it dulled my commitment to our football team. I continued to have a season ticket and attend the home games – now with Ingrid, Jack and Ben, and their friend Michele. Over the years we had distributed our combined adoration amongst some of Arsenal's biggest stars – Thierry Henry, Robert Pires, Emmanuel Petit, Freddie Ljungberg.

Now, in this 'charity of the season' year, at every home game, we would gaze in wonder as the massive screens at each end of the pitch broadcast a specially made TreeHouse appeal video. Larger than life, here were images of Danny and his mates, streaming out to the 60,000 people in the stadium.

On the day of the visit, it rained. And rained. And rained. Much of the planned visit required time outdoors, for endless photographs with the children in the playground, and then – while sporting hard hats and fluorescent-yellow tabards – Arsène and the players stood on the muddy building site of what would one day be TreeHouse's permanent home. With immense good grace, they did not try to curtail these out-of-doors duties nor show any sign of impatience and discomfort in the downpour. The rain ruined Arsène's jacket, such that a member of the PR team had to advise that he remove it before appearing in front of the TV cameras at the Sky Sports press conference.

About me, I remember only a 'this is not happening' sensation, a simultaneous mix of disbelief and hero-worship. The photos of the press conference, at which I sat next to Arsène, suggest I managed to disguise the potential to explode that

Linda had identified. I appear stunned and solemn – tran-
quilised, you might think. But the more informal photos of me
showing Arsène round the school are hilariously different. I'm
kind of swooning, kind of starstruck. The caption Michele
suggested was, 'Oh Arsène, can I lick your shoes?'

I loved that day then and I love it now. And it wasn't even a
one-off. There would be more visits from more players
(Fàbregas, Gallas) and more visits from Arsène.

The final visit was at the formal opening of our completed
new building. With Trevor Pears (our wonderful philan-
thropic supporter) and Ed Balls (the then Secretary of State
for Children, Schools and Families), Arsène officially launched
the Pears National Centre for Autism Education. A tour of
the centre featured a session in the new sports hall, where
Arsène kicked a football around with some of the children.
Richard Hatter and I watched, both of us awed and enthralled
by how far our charity had come. Richard supports Spurs, so
I think he took a special delight in the spectacle of Arsène
deliberately missing a save, so that a TreeHouse pupil could
score a goal.

What was particularly enchanting about this whole episode
was the glorious obliviousness of most of the pupils. Danny is
familiar with the Arsenal logo – it's on his bedding and his
backpack and some of his clothes – and he's grown up with
televised football matches being constantly broadcast in both
parents' homes. He has even attended a few matches. The first
was a great success, being a reserve match with a small and quiet
crowd. The final one – a noisy Premier League confrontation
– brought about a despairing meltdown.

But regardless of these mixed experiences of Arsenal, one
thing I know for sure is that Danny is untouched by the
concept of fame and team allegiance. I don't think he has any
notion of taking sides, or judging people on account of their
inbuilt loyalties, their likes and dislikes, their ideologies and

their enmities. So when these feted international superstars came to visit, they were just ordinary, entirely unremarkable young men. The vast gulf of fame and money and status between spectacular football stars and the TreeHouse children was irrelevant to him.

26

The Queen

Two days after my fiftieth birthday, I received a letter telling me that I had been recommended for an OBE in recognition of my 'voluntary services to autistic children'. This was unexpected! I didn't know whether to laugh or cry. I swore a lot. I thought how amused my late father would have been, given our political differences and my rather militant history. But I decided to accept the honour in any case, and I still smile when I think of our motley crew being given VIP treatment in Buckingham Palace.

We turn up in a rather battered Renault and are ushered into the interior car park, inhabited by rows of classy upmarket vehicles – Rolls-Royces, Mercedes, Jags. Two uniformed and smiling attendants greet us, ready and waiting with a wheelchair for my mother (obviating the need to unfold and haul hers from the boot of the car). We enter through a side door and I immediately exclaim, 'Danny, you're *inside Buckingham Palace!*' And of course this means nothing to him whatsoever, which is exactly why this is such fun.

He had been in pain overnight, and it is only thanks to tramadol and his favourite toy Slinky that he is here, with Corey, my mother and my sister Jane, to witness my attempts at a curtsy and a conversation with the Queen. We have been permitted a fourth guest on account of Danny's need for a carer, thereby honouring the legislation around 'reasonable adjustments' for disability.

Arrangements have been made to ensure that my guests are seated in a place that will allow a rapid escape, in case Danny gets upset, or indulges one time too many in his favourite ritual – hurling his Slinky across the floor, then jumping up and down with a happy whoop before picking it up. Thus my group occupies the very best seats in the huge ballroom – front row, looking straight up to where the Queen will honour her subjects. It means that after the ceremony, Danny will be in central view when Her Majesty walks down the aisle and exits. A lady-in-waiting will come up to Jane to tell her that Her Majesty enquired as to the well-being of the autistic boy. Danny didn't wonder at all about the Queen, but the Queen asked about Danny.

I trust it was not the first time an autistic teenager with severe intellectual impairment had been welcomed into this most grand and elevated of places, but even so, it was important that such an event should not be a one-off. I felt that Danny's presence – and his obliviousness to its meaning – conveyed a strong levelling message about equality and human diversity in all its forms. I recognised with gratitude that the way we were treated reflected a welcoming attitude that, I chose to believe, came right from the person at the very top.

27

DINAH

How lucky this was: on a cold, grey weekend afternoon, to be walking with Danny along Blackstock Road, on our way back from the shop that sold plastic rainbow-coloured Slinky toys; to see a tall, striking, middle-aged woman on the corner by the push-button crossing; to walk past but then remember just in time who I think she might be, and so turn back.

Later, she will tell me that her first thought was, 'Aha, an autistic boy', and that it was Danny who made her stop at the very point at which I too was turning back.

'Excuse me, are you Dinah Murray?' I asked. I introduced Danny and myself. 'We've only met once before, I think, but you also sent me a lovely text.' And then on the spur of the moment I added: 'We live really near, would you like to come back to ours for a cup of tea?'

Dr Dinah Murray was one of the co-authors of the 1998 literature review of autism educational interventions that had led to Su's and my first meeting with officials and academics at the DfEE.[1] Dinah was not at that original meeting, but her name stayed fixed in my mind because of the frequency with which I would look at the pale-blue tome and reference it in campaign and policy documents.

Several years later, I met her in person when she attended a meeting of the Advisory Group for the All Party Parliamentary Group on Autism. She and colleagues were spearheading a campaign against overuse of medication on autistic patients, under the acronym APANA.[2]

I heard again about Dinah via Debbie Storey, whose campaign brought her into contact with several prominent people within the autism movement.

'I had an email from Dinah Murray,' Debbie had said, almost in hushed tones, implying the impressive reach of her influence, as if she had said: 'I *even* had an email from Dinah Murray.'

My own equivalent of Debbie's pleasure at hearing from Dinah came after I had contributed an article in a popular newspaper about why I couldn't imagine wanting to cure Danny of his autism. I received a text from Dinah, warmly supportive of what I had written.

But still we did not meet or communicate further, until the Blackstock Road/Brownswood Road junction found us together in the same place at the same time.

What better way to connect than to sit and chat over a cup of tea at the kitchen table, with Danny watching his videos and demolishing his latest Slinky? He would bend, chew and break the Slinky rapidly, leaving small strands of coloured plastic all over the floor. I derived a perverse enjoyment at seeing the rainbow strands strewn on the pavement near to the car. You could trace his movements, like Hansel and Gretel, via the Slinky trail. Though to my shame I'm not sure that I always picked them up, so some poor Islington street-cleaner probably did not find Danny's mess as charming as I did.

After that first meeting with Dinah, a friendship grew, year on year. We met members of each other's families, we invited each other to gatherings, we shared our love of Kurt Vonnegut and of dancing alone in the kitchen, and we discussed and debated along the way.

★

It is chiefly thanks to Dinah that I would meet many leading autistic thinkers and campaigners in the UK and abroad. She introduced me to Dr Wenn Lawson, whose emphasis on 'diffability' as opposed to 'disability' encapsulates the spirit in which difference is to be respected and accommodated rather than shunned and demonised.[3] And it was through Dinah that I was able to make direct contact with Michelle Dawson.

Imagine how it was for Dinah and me when we touched upon the painful topic of ABA – about which we had such contrasting thoughts and feelings. It is probably fair to say that we both inwardly imploded when we talked about this together, so linked was it to our belief systems. Sometimes we skirted around the subject, sometimes we dared to tackle it. We tried to find common ground where we could. And it was this – the desire to understand and find common ground – that made Dinah so special. She was open enough to visit TreeHouse, to see for herself rather than rely on rumour as the basis of her opinions.

Her visit was probably more enlightening for me than it was for her. Granted, I think she appreciated that the children weren't having their autism battered out of them, that the goals on the curriculum seemed relevant and constructive, that the atmosphere was kind and celebratory. But the repetition entailed in some of the learning tasks that she observed was not for her, and nor was the intensive face-to-face teaching that was common. (I should add that this was not uniform for all the pupils. Some moved on to work independently, in a way that might not look like the stereotypical ABA at all. Subtle and 'higher level' ABA is indeed *totally* different in appearance, but few detractors know this.)

'Put it this way,' she said. 'I would not have learned anything if I'd been taught that way.'

This really struck home.

Because, I realised, I wouldn't have wanted to be taught that way either, at least not after the age of about three.

Not having a learning disability and not having difficulties in processing information delivered in words, I became comfortable at a young age with group teaching, and later with lectures and independent, solitary study. The last thing I would have wanted, I think, at any age beyond pre-school, would have been the approach that was being adopted towards some of the pupils in the TreeHouse classrooms.

And this, I believe, is where the great divide begins. For those autistic people who received inflexible forms of ABA and found it ghastly – and for many neurotypical onlookers – it is hard to imagine that anyone might feel differently about this intensity of approach to teaching and learning, particularly if it continues into school-age settings.

It would take me a long time to figure this out.

In the end I would come to reconcile these views about ABA, for autistics and learning-disabled people and neurotypicals alike, by reaffirming the important message that 'one size does not fit all'. In Danny's case, as for other children at TreeHouse, one had to factor in the reality of intellectual disability, as well as nuances of personality differences and learning style. Left to his own devices he would have enjoyed his videos and his stimmy toys until his dying day, but without TreeHouse's intervention in teaching him to use his communication book, for example, or to request a break when things were getting too much, his life would have been much narrower, he would have had much less agency to make choices, to convey his wishes and his needs. For Danny, the individualised approach, with prompts and fine-tuned responses from his tutors, suited him perfectly. Add to that the issue of personality. Danny is inherently sociable and affectionate, he enjoys building relationships with familiar people, so the permanent presence of a teacher or support worker was a positive experience for him.

But it was Dinah's observation that helped me think all of this through. Until then I hadn't fully appreciated this aspect of the opposition to ABA.

Dinah also took the trouble to send me her notes about our great divide. She could acknowledge, for example, that the emphasis on using data to identify both progress and barriers to learning might be very useful in helping a tutor adapt their approach accordingly. She could see the value of personalising the curriculum and identifying the uniquely individual motivations of each child. And she could recognise that the atmosphere was not in any way punitive. She would later describe this as a 'jolly attitude' and 'nicey-nice ABA'.[4]

And this too was a crucial eye-opener for me. I was finally coming to appreciate the extent to which much of the attitudinal climate towards autism had been negative, pathologizing, damaging – for decade upon decade – and how this was devastating to generations of autistic people. I had struggled to appreciate this fully until now, because as far as I could tell, the autistic children I knew were all on the receiving end of unconditional parental love and kind professionals. But beyond my immediate circle – out there in the realm of many scientists and ABA 'hardliners' – I gradually became aware of how toxic the sense of disapproval, distaste, even repulsion, about autistic people's failure to be 'normal' could be.

'Someone asked me if I feel proud to be autistic,' Dinah once told me. She continued: 'I said to them, "How could I feel proud, when everything I hear about autism tells me I'm broken, I'm inadequate, I'm impaired?"'

She felt like this, despite everything she achieved and everything she was.

On another occasion, we were talking about a particularly damaging interaction between an autistic patient and a (renowned) psychiatrist.

'He doesn't love autistic people,' she concluded.

Aha.

We hope that anyone working in a 'helping profession' will feel well-disposed towards their clients, pupils, patients. If they can't love them, we hope they will like them, and if they don't like them, we hope they will at least behave as if they do. When you're working with a child, in particular, you should be on their side. Dinah was telling me that all too often, autistic people – *even small children* – have felt that their so-called helpers aren't on their side.

To receive this sense of disapproval, day in, day out, must surely be unbearable. And so, to mete it out – however unconsciously – must surely be some kind of abuse.

28

THE WRIGHTS AND RIGHTS

In 2008, Bob and Suzanne Wright, the controversial but powerful founders of the American charity Autism Speaks, were invited to the UK.

As part of their tour, they visited TreeHouse, and Bob Wright was invited to deliver the inaugural TreeHouse annual lecture. I explained to Ian Wiley, then TreeHouse chief executive, that this invitation was so contentious and provocative among the autism rights community in the UK that we might even 'need bouncers on the door'. Probably an exaggeration, but not far off. I sought Dinah's advice and introduced her to Ian.

Another person might have refused to do business with TreeHouse, would have 'let the behaviourists stew,' as she later mentioned to me privately.[1] But Dinah helped turn the event into an opportunity to publicise the discourse around different wings of the autism movement. At that point, Autism Speaks was wedded to a vision of cure and prevention of autism without appreciating the offence this mission, promoted with unsophisticated zeal, might cause at least to some.[2]

So, in the interests of balance, TreeHouse funded Dinah to produce a film made by autistic people and about autistic people, a film which would be shown on a loop at the reception accompanying the TreeHouse lecture. It is *Something About Us* and is available on YouTube.[3] The lecture led the *Daily Telegraph* to publish an article about contrasting perspectives on autism, in which Anya Ustaszewski was quoted with the most succinct and powerful of autism-as-identity sayings:

If you take away my autism you take away me.[4]

As simple as that, reflecting what Donna and Paul and I had shared between us all those years before, and which had crystallised as a certainty during my depression.

On the night of the lecture, several friends and acquaintances, including Ingrid and Larry, were among the audience in the London Assembly council chamber. I was a panel member alongside Anya and Bob Wright. Jon Snow was chairman for an inevitably challenging event to manage – what with the heckling and the polar opposite viewpoints gathered there and expressed forcefully from the floor.

The most powerful interjection came from Larry, whom you can see in the recording of the event on the Rightful Lives website.[5] You can also see Anya, responding eloquently and convincingly to Bob, who is enthusiastic about looking for a cure for autism. Anya counter-proposes that if you seek to prevent or cure autism, you are seeking a world where there are no more autistic people, something that would be as harmful to all as it is insulting to autistics. What is needed is an endeavour to help autistic people be the best autistic person they can be, not a mission to eliminate autistic people from society.

It is my job to be the third speaker. At one point I talk about the issue of suffering. Some people want to prevent or cure autism, I reckon, because they genuinely believe that autism equates with greater-than-average suffering (relative to being neurotypical). That is when Larry shouts in an impassioned cry:

'*Suffering is a basic condition of humanity, there is nobody who has not suffered in some way or other.*'

Autistic suffering, he was suggesting, is the kind of suffering that minorities go through when they are oppressed, and the remedy is to tackle the oppression, not the victim. In contrast, other forms of suffering are common to us all.

Here we are, then. The crux of what would become my doctoral thesis. What are the ethical implications regarding the rationale for preventing, or indeed terminating, a pregnancy on the grounds of disability? Which kinds of suffering do we try to prevent, and which kinds do we see as inevitable – and even, perhaps, opportunities through which we can grow? For many people, existing in our inequitable world comes with daily challenges.

Is trying to prevent the birth of a disabled person any different from trying to prevent the birth of someone because they will encounter poverty? Echo that for being born into any state of relative social disadvantage – such as being born female, or gay, in many parts of the world. Echo that more loudly for the sections of the world's population who live in war zones, or under totalitarian regimes. Yes, you could argue that disability and neurodivergence place additional burdens that even an ideal society could not entirely ameliorate. While this may be true (for example, see Wharmby's account of some of the interior challenges of being autistic[6]), it is still far from clear that they are so problematic as to justify withholding support or preventing the possibility of existence.

So when we think of disability, if we put all our eggs in the 'prevention/cure' basket, rather than the 'individual support and radical societal change' basket, isn't that rather like saying, 'You'll never stop homophobic hate crime, so let's prevent the birth of all gay people'?

Or how about: 'You'll never stop male violence against women, so let's only have boys' – or perhaps: 'You'll never stop male violence full stop, so let's only have girls'? These examples are extreme of course, but for those who regard the suffering of disabled people as *primarily* about social disadvantage and cultural norms, and only secondarily (if at all) about medical prognosis, these analogies are – I believe -- illuminating. We need to be extremely careful to distinguish between the kinds of suffering we should prevent through medical and other individually targeted interventions and the kinds of suffering caused by injustice and cruelty, or indeed ignorance and misunderstanding. They require radically different initiatives, and widely differing attitudes towards the 'sufferer'. And in any case, what is the rationale for making a categorical distinction between people who need support from a very young age, as opposed to all of us who will need support at some time in our lives?

Larry's interjection spoke volumes about the ethical challenges we face, all of us humans who are thinking about what kinds of lives are good and worthwhile, what kinds of lives are intolerable, and what role, if any, medical science should have in determining what kinds of people are welcome in our world – who should be born, and who should not. I couldn't do other than be glad for his interruption, even though there was no time to respond adequately.

'Society disables us more than autism ever could,' Anya said. This hints at an important midway perspective: regardless of how you feel about autism, the best thing you can do is to address the wider oppressions that are externally imposed. It's more important to address our social and cultural environment than to go down the rabbit warren of esoteric genomic exploration.

The Wrights were gracious about what must have felt like a pummelling.

And later, Dinah would say that the TreeHouse support was immaculate in terms of autism-friendly organisation and helpfulness. I felt enormously proud of and grateful towards my colleagues, and so glad Dinah gave this feedback, which was typical of her desire to give credit and seek out the positive – particularly in circumstances where others would in contrast highlight the areas of divergence.

This ability to seek out common ground and build bridges between people who might otherwise be at loggerheads, and to do so without compromising either her fundamental allegiances and beliefs or her ability to speak her mind, is not what you might call a 'typical' autistic strength. And I should add that this ability of Dinah's is one that is sorely lacking in many of the neurotypicals who dominate our world. It was a quality that rescued our friendship five years later.

In 2013, a documentary programme about ABA was scheduled to be aired on BBC 4,[7] and in response the producers of the topical TV magazine show *The Wright Stuff* decided it would be fun to stage a prior studio discussion. I agreed to participate. But by the time I was sitting waiting to go on, it seemed like a terrible idea. The caption headlining the item was '*Cure for autism? Treat children like dogs!*' In my wildest imaginings, I couldn't have envisaged such a crude, jaw-dropping shocker of a headline. So, distancing myself from the goal of cure, I first tried to explain what ABA was in a way that broadened it out from dog training, saying that it was underpinned by scientific principles that operate far beyond the domain of autism. When pressed, I said that it could be 'incredibly positive'. I still believe this, but I know it would be equally honest to say that ABA can be 'incredibly negative' – depending crucially on how it is defined, for what purpose it is applied, on the values and attitudes and skills of the practitioners, and on the needs and learning style of the individual. None of these caveats, all of which needed further elucidation, felt possible in a short TV slot.

Dinah couldn't bring herself to watch it, because she knew how upsetting she would find it. But later, after various emails whose details I don't remember, she wrote me this:

Dear one.
It's OK.
It's all about love.

And yes, should this not be what lies underneath our beliefs and our conflicts? Surely, beneath the despair at warring views on how the world should be, there lies in most of us a desire to do the right thing with and by our fellow humans? Are we not burning with shared questions, such as: how are we to be in the world? And what concessions do we have to make, to and for one another, to maintain some kind of inclusive future for us all? Who do we listen to? Who do we believe? And what do we do with contradictory information, narratives and allegiances? And when should we agree to disagree, in order to pursue a greater imperative to promote our human connectedness?

Postscript

Dinah died in July 2021. I, like so many others who praised her stellar contribution in the field of autism, wanted also to testify to her less public influence – her loyalty, support and friendship, her sensitivity and her kindness, her commitment to justice and her wonderful sense of humour.

And with Dinah in mind, it feels important to take you to the words of a man who, in his teens, was diagnosed with Asperger syndrome:

I think there is more in common between people who have autism and people who do not than we sometimes acknowledge. This is not due to there being a bit of autism in most of us, as is sometimes suggested. Rather, this is due to there being a lot of human in all of us.[8]

29

GROUNDHOG YEARS

31 December 2007

New Year's Eve. I lie awake and contemplate the coming year. I face two seemingly insurmountable challenges.

First: how am I ever going to undertake research, and then say all the things I want to say? I hope to start working on my doctorate in 2008, but from where will I find the inspiration or the time?

And, more pressingly: how am I going to get Danny safely through adolescence and into adulthood?

At fifteen, Danny's health is no better, and the violence with which he expresses his pain and distress is becoming dangerous, for him and for me. For several years Danny has been in and out of hospital. And at home, the dents in walls from his head-butts are indelible reminders of his distress.

★

John and Sarah started to provide cover on alternate Friday evenings and Saturday mornings, and thereby make Danny's times at Nick's house safe and consequently feasible. Meanwhile, when Danny was with me, it became harder and harder to ensure either his or my safety. But just when things started to look impossible, Corey came to live with us Monday to Friday. He had been working with Danny after school for eight years, had joined us on excursions and holidays, but we had never contemplated his moving in. And yet, just when we needed him most, Corey needed a place to stay. So he took over our spare room, and enabled our fragile arrangement to continue. Danny was unable to overpower Corey physically, but of far greater significance was the deepening of mutual trust and love that had long characterised their relationship. Now, they really were like brothers.

With three of us in the house, meeting Danny's need for round-the-clock support was viable. Even so, during Corey's absence at weekends, Danny and I were alone and in effect under house arrest. I could not safely protect Danny or myself, or other members of the community if he had a meltdown outside the home. I would berate myself for not advocating convincingly enough for urgent medical attention.

Nevertheless, there were some lovely days, in which Danny seemed so well that I thought perhaps I had been over-dramatising. At these times we would go out, or have Ingrid and the boys round. They were the constants among a small handful of friends who understood our predicament – and who kept coming round anyway, to watch a televised Arsenal match or an episode of *Strictly Come Dancing*.

31 December 2008

New Year's Eve again. It had been another tough Christmas. Danny and I beat the now familiar path to the Royal Free. Once more, we found ourselves on the children's ward, ninth floor, in a room overlooking a panoramic view spanning miles of north-east London.

I remember the relief, the total relief, of being in hospital. For a while, decision-making could be handed over to the medical and nursing teams; for a while, I could stop trying to pretend that life could in any way be 'normal'.

It seemed to be permanently nighttime, and it felt as if we were on a spaceship, the starship *Enterprise*, powering its way through the silent universe, lights blazing through the darkness. The only place in the endless void of space where people were living, breathing, working, moving was this tall hospital building. The world outside the hospital vanished; we and this army of helping people were the only living souls. Sealed inside the spaceship, Danny and I could surrender to our helplessness, within the safe machinery of the hospital that murmured and thrummed through the day and night, its momentum and focus guarding us against the vast meaningless emptiness beyond.

Safety and hope returned, thanks in part to 'heroic' doses of oral laxative and a series of enemas, and thanks, too, to the New Year's Eve visit of Corey, Ingrid, Michele and Su. They smuggled in cava and supper, we toasted one another, and Danny giggled while Corey pressed various buttons on the bed, making it rise and fall like a gentle fairground ride.

Corey and Ingrid were still there at midnight when, all over London, hundreds of fireworks displays lit the sky. Wave upon wave of colour and light transformed the night, and we gazed in wonder for what felt like hours across a wide illuminated landscape of tower blocks and low-rise houses, interspersed with parks and trees, undulating across the miles towards the distant horizon.

The next morning, Nick and Amanda, with their boys Lowell and Jesse, came to visit. It was a cheerful New Year family gathering, unusual for being in a hospital and for being the six of us together, and it was all rather fun for its novelty and for the renewed hope that Danny was on the mend. The unbidden beauty of the previous night's fireworks display, this treat that had unexpectedly come to us alongside the misfortune of being hospitalised, clearly chimed with Nick. It inspired the lyrics of a song he later co-wrote with Ben Folds.[1]

And so it goes, that the ripples from our lives make their way to unexpected places and to unknown people.

★

The temporary relief of this happy day did not continue over the following months. Again and again, doctors would encourage us to reduce the laxatives, arguing that it may be an excess of them that was causing Danny pain. And again and again these attempts to reduce the dose would merely exacerbate the problem. He was on regular opiate-based pain-control medication, which we knew entailed a vicious circle because of its constipating effects, not to mention the danger of addiction, yet without which he was in serious danger of giving himself brain damage from repeatedly banging his head against hard surfaces. The other danger was that he might cause serious injury to me and to others as he lashed out in desperation, not just for a few minutes but protractedly, hour after hour.

Days and days were spent in a hot bath, one of the only places he could get relief. Nighttimes, too: his gut was no respecter of the need to sleep, and sometimes things were worse at night, perhaps because of the reflux caused by lying down, perhaps because of spasms induced by being horizontal. He would be in a deep sleep and then suddenly sit bolt upright, screaming, hitting his head with the back of his hand or leaning backwards, banging it repeatedly against his bedroom wall.

The good times were all based on periods of better health for Danny. We also depended on the dedication and tireless professionalism and love of his team of carers, all at that stage privately funded by Nick.

I was not oblivious to the hard fact that I was luckier than many others who have a disabled, ill child. We were immensely, incalcu- lably fortunate that Sarah, Corey and John stayed the course, through decade after tough decade. There will not be enough people like them to go round until the status and reward for work like theirs is dramatically improved – until the whole profession is reformed. And this in turn requires a broader rethink about which roles in society we truly value, as opposed to the roles that are rewarded most generously in our current economic system.

Summer 2009

Danny underwent a colonic transit test. After eating a bowl of baked beans imbued with some radioactive substance to enable them to light up in an X-ray, he was strapped to an X-ray table mattress, to prevent his moving while images were taken (he did not understand the request to lie still). He was given lots of his favourite toys, and soothed by Corey and me either side of him, to the accompaniment of his favourite music. It was a day we had dreaded. How on earth would he stay still? How on earth would he accept being confined in this way?

As so, so often, what you dread most turns out to be OK, while the bad things that happen are what you'd never even imagined. Danny was a cooperative sweetie. He seemed to enjoy the X-ray, smiling his way through the whole procedure, which had to be repeated regularly so that they could plot how far down the gut the baked beans had travelled.

The results?

'Grossly abnormal.'

I asked the doctor to repeat what he had just told us. I was so accustomed to medical people telling me that there was no serious problem with Danny's gut that I thought I must have misheard.

'Grossly abnormal.'

It seems perverse, but I was pleased. In fact I wanted to punch the air in relief.

At last. A consultant telling us what we had struggled so hard to convey. Instead of downplaying our reports and our painstaking data and ignoring our pleas for help, here was a medical authority acknowledging that there was something significantly awry about Danny's gastrointestinal tract. Such vindication was sweet news, going some way to banish the self-doubts and inward self-interrogation that had plagued me and taken up precious energy in the previous years.

Of course the gross abnormality was not in itself good news. It presaged more pain, further tests, various intrusive attempts to deal with the problem. We knew the score. And we knew that yet again we needed to widen the pool of supportive people.

30

LEE

Lee is a key person whose singular contribution to the lives of Nick, Danny and me is such that he gets his own section in two different books.

In Nick's book *31 Songs*,[1] Lee was the man who fed Nick's voracious musical appetite, and in so doing became a good friend. It is not really a competition of course, but I now claim a superior and even more significant role for Lee.

The first meeting between Danny and Lee came about because Danny expressed the need to pee. It was maybe 1998; Danny was five years old. We had gone on a bus ride, Danny and me, into Islington. Public transport was usually fun – he liked being on the move and tapping on the windows, and when we reached our stop we would go to a café and he would enjoy a bag of crisps and a drink. On this particular day, while we were walking along Upper Street, back to the bus stop for our return journey home, Danny said, 'Dee.'

One of the few words Danny had acquired and retained was 'dee', his word for toilet (and also for train).

'Train all gone,' I said. 'Bus.'

'Dee, dee,' Danny replied with more urgency.

'Show me the sign, Danny.'

He touched his shoulder, which was his approximation for the Makaton sign for toilet, not train.

Uh-oh. If we retraced our steps to the café, this would (I knew from previous experience) elicit great distress, a meltdown. If we proceeded to the bus, even if Danny managed to hold it in, there would be a crescendoing clamour for 'dee', with accompanying agitation, and maybe he would wet his pants in the bargain. Best avoid that too.

Where to find a loo?

Lee's shop. There was Lee's music shop. I had met Lee maybe just once before, and rather briefly. But he would understand, and be utterly relaxed and unfazed by the immediacy, the no-small-talk, no-polite-preamble, 'Hello, Danny needs to use your toilet' nature of the demand. It was the perfect start to Danny's and my relationship with Lee. When our contact resumed many years later, there would never have to be social niceties; there would always be authentic cut-the-crap interaction.

What happened was this: as Nick's chapter had foretold, Lee's shop finally became the casualty of an industrial revolution. CDs were increasingly bought on the internet, and later still they made way for music that was downloaded or streamed directly. With two children to bring up, Lee's need for an alternative source of income forced him to enter a profession towards which he felt, let us say, ambivalent. He became an estate agent.

But this was great for me because Lee's office was in Muswell Hill, and we started to meet occasionally for lunch. These meetings became little islets of comfort. We shared confidences about our tortured, tangled personal lives and we made each other laugh.

During the first years of our friendship, Lee sometimes witnessed directly, and sometimes heard me describe, the smashed mirrors and dented walls, the bruises and scratches on my hands and forearms – all brought about by Danny's pain.

'I hate admitting it,' I sobbed in one tearful phone call, 'but sometimes I am frightened of my own son.'

'You know it's not safe for him to stay with you much longer,' Lee said. 'He's getting stronger. He could seriously injure you.'

'But he can't go to residential school,' I sobbed some more.

'Yes, he can.'

'No, no.'

'Yes, Virginia. Yes.'

'No,' I wailed. 'No, no, no.'

Lee stayed on the phone while I cried and cried.

Danny going away was unthinkable. I would be heartbroken, and guilt-ridden. The thought of him missing home, feeling vulnerable and rejected and with no ability to understand what had brought about this separation was unbearable. But it wasn't these imaginings that stopped me giving it consideration. Indeed I could see the arguments in favour, since I knew of other families for whom, despite similar heartfelt fears and emotions, residential school had proved essential and beneficial, instances where the children had thrived and the families had regathered their depleted energies and rebuilt their hopes, where attachments and bonds had remained intact and even grown stronger. If Danny hadn't been unwell, I might seriously have explored the possibility of a waking-hour curriculum in an integrated residential care and education setting, in which dedicated workers would support him round the clock, providing consistency, stimulus, expertise, care.

But Danny's medical problems made everything different. I couldn't imagine any staff team – however marvellous – having the dedication, or know-how, or 24/7 precision, backed up by years of knowing Danny and previous nursing experience, to make daily judgements on levels of laxative, types of painkiller, when to give him a break from eating, when to push fluids, when to re-examine the data to find potential correlations between diet, behaviour, pain, pain relief, bowel movements.

I was too distraught to explain all this at the time, and Lee stayed quiet and supportive through my tears. He never mentioned sending Danny away again.

Instead, he did something glorious.

He became one of Danny's care team.

At the point when Lee decided he could face being an estate agent no longer, work with Danny was waiting for him. Not only would he do the home run from school every afternoon (freeing up some time for me to pursue charity and research commitments), but also he would be on hand to assist with what had by then become a ghastly daily routine. This involved administering rectal enemas as the only way to alleviate Danny's constipation and his pain, and it needed at least two people, because understandably Danny fought to avoid the restraint and the gross intrusion.

Danny always forgave us afterwards, with a return of smiles and good cheer, happy with the relief that the enema usually brought. And he became very attached to Lee, often burying his head in Lee's chest in order to receive soothing head massages, or stretching his legs over Lee's lap as they sat together on a sofa.

We devised a traffic-lights system. Whenever I was on my own with Danny, Lee agreed to have his phone on at all times of the day and night. If I texted 'Green', it meant all was well. If I texted 'Yellow' it meant 'we might need you to get in the car and come and help us any minute now'. 'Red' meant 'whatever you're doing, stop it now and get here ASAP'. He lived fifteen minutes away, and so I knew – and Nick knew – that however bad things were, help would soon be at hand.

As if all this wasn't lucky enough, Lee gave us two more gifts.

He decided I needed a partner, and found one for me. I could see no hope of ever meeting someone who would find anything attractive about a depleted, autism- and GI-dysfunction-obsessed fifty-year-old woman. A woman whose life revolved around a delightful but chronically unwell and sometimes-violent young man. A woman whose nights were usually disrupted, and who on her nights off was usually exhausted.

Lee decided to take matters into his own hands. He set up a *Guardian* Soulmates profile for me,[*] gave me an alias, wrote the blurb about me and selected a photo (for only interested parties to see). When I had one week left of the month's trial, and had done nothing, followed up no one, Lee came round one evening, forced me to choose five potential dates, and suggested wording which I was persuaded to email to all five. I was sceptical but helpless in the face of his concern and his determination. He would later explain to Nick and Amanda that he bullied me into it.

Of the five we picked out, there was one who seemed way out of my league but who Lee had already decided was my best bet. It was not just this man's physical appearance – though that was nice; it was the things he had written in his profile and the way he expressed himself. It seemed he was warm and kind and enthusiastic and creative. He was looking for someone who would share weekends with him and his teenage sons.

'Well that's not going to work for a start,' I protested. 'Danny and I won't be able to share weekends with two teenage boys.'

'Never mind, it's just a bit of fun.'

'But he lives in Enfield. That's quite far.' It was on the very edge of the ten-mile radius that Lee felt was the maximum realistic range.

'Just send him an email, and then ring him.'

★

---

[*] Soulmates was the *Guardian*'s online dating service. It closed in 2020 after fifteen years.

Sometime in the late spring of 2009 you could have found me sitting in a gastropub in East Finchley, feeling fed up. I was exhausted after a gruelling night with Danny, who had been in pain from 4 a.m. I resented wasting my time on this venture, and sent a grumpy text to Lee.

My date had texted me to say he was running late. Yeah yeah. But something in the final 'don't go away!' made me smile. Still grumpy and bored, I nevertheless sat and waited.

And then at long last, in he walked.

Within weeks, I was telling people excitedly about Adrian – his warmth, his energy, his originality. Nor did he appear to be disconcerted by any of my backstory, and I was thoroughly bemused.

He met Danny, and although Danny didn't immediately warm to him, he didn't push him away either.

There is one night that stands out in my memory as pivotal. Adrian had emerged from the bedroom dressed and with shoes on at 3 a.m., passing me on the landing by Danny's door where I was sitting, waiting for the painkillers to calm him down.

'Are you leaving?' I asked, numbly assuming that this was one 3 a.m. disruption too many.

'No of course not,' he laughed. 'I'm going downstairs to make you a cup of tea.'

In early September, I met Adrian's two sons, Jamie and Josh – where else but at the Emirates? A friendly football match seemed as good a place as any for a first meeting. Minimum conversation, mutual entertainment, but enough scope for checking each other out.

The moment I saw Jamie and Josh standing with their dad at Arsenal Underground station, I recognised them as older versions of the sweet little boys I had seen in photos at Adrian's home. It was as if I already knew them. I approached and they each gave me a hug, and I felt a cautious stirring of belief that this whole thing might, just, in some way or another, work.

★

Lee pulled off something my mother would later describe as a 'miracle' in finding Adrian, Jamie and Josh. And yet there is even more of Lee in the story of Danny and me that I want to explain.

It was Lee's ability to see Danny in all his loveliness, and to know Danny's strengths, that made him my soul brother. Lee took the time to discover in Danny the qualities that so many other people could not be bothered to find, or perhaps were too scared to uncover.

He did this in his singular way.

For example, while on holiday in the USA, Lee inexplicably decided to have an enema, 'out of curiosity'. I didn't ask for more details, but suffice it to say that the experience caused him to think anew how amazing and long-suffering Danny was, at that time when rectal enemas were part of his daily routine.

Then Lee trained to do voluntary work for the charity Kith & Kids.* During the training, an exercise required volunteers to try to communicate with one another without recourse to words or pictures. They could gesture, but they were not allowed to write or talk or draw. Lee was awestruck by the challenge; it was so very hard. And then he thought of the skill with which Danny had learned to convey his needs and express himself without these tools that most of us take for granted.

'Danny, you're a genius,' he exclaimed when he next saw him.

---

* Kith & Kids (www.kithandkids.org.uk) provides activities, opportunities, information and support for people with a learning disability or autism, their parents and siblings.

Another time, Lee had a knee operation and lay awake overnight in his hospital bed thinking of Danny. The general anaesthetic still in Lee's system was making it impossible for him to pass urine; his bladder muscles weren't working properly, however much he sensed the need and willed some relief. He was reminded of the fact that Danny's intestinal and bladder muscles suffer similar malfunction.

'That man's a giant, a fucking giant,' he said to me when we talked about it a few days later. He added: 'Where would we all be without him?'

Yes indeed, where? Lee was capturing the spirit of Danny's family, and all the support staff and teachers who have fallen in love with Danny over his lifetime. People who see Danny's ability to forgive, to move on, to greet the new moment without bitterness about the past. I can only wonder at this luminosity of spirit in him, be awed and admiring and proud and grateful.

There are other gems from Lee, too, texts which I savour.

'Danny is better than any of them, you realise when you get to know him …'

And then:

'But it takes time.'

This is true, I believe, of most autistic people and people with profound intellectual and communication disabilities. In a world where rapid-fire conversation or easy banter are keys to mutual entertainment, not many people trouble to take the time to see value in people who offer different qualities. I believe that in not doing so, they lose out on a potentially rich area of human connection, humour, warmth and discovery.

Another text from Lee contained Happy Birthday wishes 'to the biggest man I know'.

And perhaps my favourite, as a PS in a text about the uniqueness of Danny's different way of being:

'You can stuff neurotypical up your arse.'

Part 5

THE BIG QUESTIONS

'To wish simultaneously to celebrate a type of person and bring about their extinction is quite a moral juggling act.'

Simon Jarrett, *Community Living*

The rapid pace of change that had been a feature of previous years showed no sign of slowing down in the years that followed. We would gain, and lose, people we needed and loved. My hoped-for time for studying and writing would face setbacks. And we were heading for a crisis.

31

HELEN KEELER AND EUGENICS

Just as I was starting to study for my doctorate, along came a
book entitled *The Ethics of Autism*, written by Deborah
Barnbaum.[1] When I saw the title, I wondered if I would have
anything novel to say – maybe Barnbaum had covered all the
ground already. Dipping in, I quickly realised it was scholarly
and in many respects authoritative, steeped in academic references, citing the works of psychologists and philosophers.
Should I just give up?

In fact, a closer read of her book had precisely the opposite
effect. It was exactly what I needed to get going, because I
reacted so strongly against it. It was a necessary springboard,
giving me the impetus to plunge in at the deep end, no longer
fearful or cowed.

I disagreed with her on several points. First, she based her
concept of autism almost exclusively on the idea that autistic
people do not possess theory of mind.[2] This was despite the fact
that successor theories had by then become every bit as, or
more, persuasive,[3] and that in any case she herself acknowledged later in the book that not all autistic people do lack
theory of mind.[4] She then argued that this notion of autism
meant autistic people were not fully part of the 'moral

community' – even though this concept is a deeply ambiguous and contested area within moral philosophy. And lastly, on the basis of her assertions, she proposed that prospective parents should aim to avoid having autistic children. This might be possible if, for example, technologies ever become available to identify, and then reject, so-called 'at risk' eggs, sperm, embryos or foetuses in relation to autism.

Here, then, was Barnbaum apparently flirting with eugenics – the removal from the human gene pool of certain characteristics that are deemed to be harmful or redundant. I am open to the idea that there may be specific areas of genetic exploration that are truly valuable, even though the history of the eugenics movement is entirely repulsive. There is at least a discussion to be had about the potential of eliminating or editing genes that contribute to Huntington's or Tay-Sachs disease, or specific types of cancer.

But Barnbaum's suggestion of eugenics with regard to autism, not just as a choice for parents *but as an active moral obligation*, was astonishing to me. Her assertion relied heavily on the work of another philosopher, Joel Feinberg, who had written about the rights of children to 'an open future'.[5] Barnbaum argued that autistic children were incapable of exercising this right, because, she said, the absence of theory of mind closed off important opportunities, such as mutual and reciprocal relationships. This was despite many criticisms not only of the 'absent theory of mind' idea, but also of Feinberg's position.[6] For whose future is more 'open' – that of a child born in poverty, in a war zone, in a totalitarian state, or that of an autistic or learning-disabled child born in a wealthy country with a relatively advanced welfare system? There are multiple situations in which people have no opportunity to choose the circumstances of their lives, and whose options for autonomy and liberty once they become adults are severely constrained. Does this oblige every potential parent in such situations to stop having children? No: in my opinion, it does not.

This may all seem rather abstract, a bit like the 'angels on a pinhead' theological arguments of the Middle Ages that heralded disenchantment with the church. And some suggest that genomic research will never be able to actualise this hypothetical situation because there are so many genes and environmental factors implicated in autism.

But these arguments are not mere indulgences and imaginings. Eugenics, I discovered in 2009, was already alive and kicking in the UK with regard to autism. And I had the privilege of meeting one of the stars of the story in this regard: Helen Keeler. I would devote a section of my doctoral thesis to the questions she raised.

★

Helen came to my attention because she wanted to tell the world about her experience when trying to become an egg donor, in order to help couples who were struggling to conceive. She had been rejected by four fertility clinics in England, because one of her children had Asperger syndrome. Presumably the clinics in question considered it too risky even to offer the choice to prospective parents. And this was despite the overall shortage of eggs. The message of this decision was that it is better to be childless than to have an autistic child, and that it is better that fewer children are born than that a new, autistic child is born. They also denied prospective parents the opportunity to reach their own, autonomous decision about any apparent risk involved. I do not know if the clinic professionals truly believed that non-existence is preferable to autistic existence, but regardless of any intention, the impact was the same.

The notion of 'risk' is fundamental here, and – I believe – we are often deeply inconsistent about the risks we take, and the calculations we unconsciously make about contrasting probabilities. When it comes to antenatal choice and reproductive technologies, we seem to live in a deeply risk-averse society. In the UK we are permitted to abort on the grounds of disability even into late pregnancy – when the foetus is capable of, but denied the opportunity for, independent life.

The Down syndrome (DS) population is at the forefront of this situation, because the condition can be detected antenatally. In the UK ninety percent of DS foetuses are aborted, and campaigners point out that terminations happen in pregnancies as far advanced as thirty-seven weeks. Iceland – not known as an illiberal country – has gone even further, such that only two or three children with DS are born each year. This is despite the fact that many DS people have fulfilling lives and achieve similar milestones to genetically typical people, are loved and celebrated equally, and inspire others every bit as much or perhaps more. While I do not discount the fact that there is an enormous range of experience within DS, I challenge the idea that decisions should be based only on the negative possibilities.*

It seems that when it comes to DS, the thinking of prospective parents – and of the medical profession that advises them – is dominated by worst-case scenarios.[7] The greater-than-average chance of profound intellectual disability, early dementia and heart problems overrides everything else there is to know about a potential DS person and the life they might lead, the love they may experience, the joy and the reward.

How many parents would decide, or be actively steered, to terminate because their potential child might have a very serious car accident, or suffer at school from bullying and exam pressure (Danny was spared both of these), or acquire a drug

---

* It is important to separate this argument from that of the pro-life lobby who oppose all abortion. I should stress that I am in favour of a woman's right to choose. What I question is how some choices are inadvertently influenced by an ableist and medicalised aversion to disability.

habit (Danny is protected from access to all but prescribed drugs), and in adulthood suffer from deep job dissatisfaction or demoralising unemployment (Danny is under no pressure to earn a living) – the relatively commonly occurring problems faced by people without identifiable chromosomal differences? (Danny is also free from worry about climate change and he doesn't dread another Trump presidency.)

So Helen Keeler raised important questions about antenatal selection and the use of reproductive technology, even at a time when it was becoming more widely acknowledged that there may be strengths and advantages in Asperger syndrome. Famous autistics such as Greta Thunberg, and UK celebrities such as Chris Packham and Christine McGuinness, have helped shift public consciousness further since then. But little has happened to affect dominant views with regard to the expendability of learning-disabled lives.

Until the 1970s, the default treatment of people with a learning disability was to separate them from their families from infancy and to deny them an education. Even recently it has been considered appropriate to let them die instead of resuscitating them in the event of a heart attack.[8]

Yet this raises all kinds of questions about our values in society, and it also requires us to address whether distinctions should be made with regard to our attitudes to autism. It suggests that an autistic person is tolerated and even welcomed and celebrated *on condition that* they have a talent or a skill. But woe betide the autistic person whose achievements are too subtle or personal to be more widely understood, even if they inspire love in others.

We do not place such burdens on neurotypical persons to justify themselves before birth. We do not say we might try to prevent their existence on our planet unless they can demonstrate that they have something useful or attractive to offer. We accept that NT people will vary; we know it can be random as to how people turn out. But when it comes to divergence from the 'normal', it seems we find it acceptable to draw the line, to stop placing equal value on their (potential) life.

All the while, the message is that some lives are in a sense valid and can be seen as fully human and with full 'personhood', but that other lives (including those with severe cognitive disabilities) are not valid – they are not true persons in the fullest sense. Some philosophers have articulated this quite clearly.[9] They argue that people with profound cognitive disabilities do not have full personhood, and/or that their moral status is no different from that of animals.

Disability campaigners hear the eugenics message loud and clear. It is this:

'We don't want more people like you in the world. And furthermore, we are going to expend a lot of money on clinical research and practice to make sure people like you will one day no longer exist.'

32

Ingrid

In 2010, when he was approaching his seventeenth birthday, Danny underwent surgery. The operation involved inserting a tube into the left side of his abdomen, through which we could administer enemas. Instead of being held down to receive a rectal enema, he would now be able to sit on the toilet, and even assist us, while we flushed the tube in his side with large volumes of enema solution, thereby bringing on a bowel movement.

Another hospital this time: the Chelsea and Westminster. Another side room off a children's ward. Another vigil, and on this occasion Danny wanted me to lie with him, squashed inside the single bed and kept in by the side bars, my arm reaching over his tummy to hold him to me. If I adjusted my position, he would pull my arm back tightly over him. Corey slept alongside us on a mattress on the floor, and periodically we would swap places.

I remember during all of this hospital stay the daily texts from Danny's Auntie Gill. Supportive, encouraging, sympathetic texts of solidarity and love. I remember Adrian dropping by regularly, all the way from his home in Enfield, and being the person to help hold Danny down for his final rectal enema, the night before the operation. And I remember missing Ingrid, who was away with the boys, staying with friends in Spain. I was longing to tell her all about it, just as I had told her about all our previous sojourns in hospitals.

But this was something I was never able to do, and to this day I dream of finding her and catching up with all the news. And then I wake up, only to know once again the impossibility of that.

★

It was the day after Arsenal had thrilled us all with their 6–0 win at the first match of the season at the Emirates, soon after Danny had finally come home from hospital.

Corey and I had put Danny to bed, and were sitting outside in the fading evening light, reflecting with relief that things seemed at last to be calm and heading in the right direction.

The phone rang and it was Ingrid, saying she had been feeling ill all day.

I suspect that another writer would somehow produce the right words for the ensuing fortnight, in a way that is honest and honourable and loving. But such a task is beyond me. Instead, all I can offer is a pitiful list, as follows:

Ambulance.

A&E.

University College Hospital.

National Hospital, Queen Square, for surgery to stem a haemorrhage in her brain.

More surgery.

Intensive Care.

Jack dashing back from the Reading Festival, running from the station through the pouring rain.

Ben leaning into Hugh's chest and weeping.

Ingrid's brothers arriving from South Africa, straight from
the airport to the hospital, for her last morning.
  Goodbyes.

★

During Ingrid's final stay in hospital, I had woken in the night and,
immediately recognising the grief of the landscape ahead, I heard a
voice in my head that said, simply and clearly, 'I can't do this alone.'
  What was this '*this*'?
  It was my whole life, my existence, the struggle for and with
Danny, the efforts to campaign, to research, the whole mixed
package of this thing that constituted my life's work and my
heart's endeavour of love for friends and family. Ingrid's friendship had held me up ever since our first meeting at the antenatal class. She had been my ally in all aspects of my and Danny's
life – autism/learning disability/SEN, Arsenal, politics, overlapping friends, interests and escapes (holidays, dancing, the
local café, gossip, laughter). She had in turn included us in the
life she led with Jack and Ben, making it possible for Danny
and me to enjoy a semblance of what typical families often
take for granted: getting together at weekends and in school
holidays, jointly celebrating birthdays, hanging out in one
another's homes and keeping abreast of each other's latest news.
  In the middle of the night I realised how lonely I felt, and
that without Ingrid it would be hard to go on.

★

I wrote this in my journal, in May 2011, nine months after
Ingrid's death:

  In the bright sunshine and to the sounds of rustling leaves in
  the wind and the babbling water fountain in the pond by

which the headstone was placed, Ingrid's ashes were laid to rest.

Her stone was embossed with the Arsenal insignia, the bright assertive red gun. She would have laughed at its eccentricity and boldness, its fidelity to her own loyalty and a jaunty defiance of gloom.

'I don't know what to say,' I said to one of Ingrid's cousins.

'There is nothing to say,' she replied. 'We come, we stay for a while, we go.'

33

Light and Shadow

The year with Adrian had been good. I saw him twice, maybe three times a week, and gradually got to know his boys. But until that point in the middle of the night when I faced my loneliness, I hadn't been relying on them. Now, though, I felt that life without them would be impossible.

Happily, they did not challenge this realisation, but rather welcomed it. They responded with grace and enthusiasm, in a way that typifies their warm natures, their instinctive talent for human connection. They had seen the challenges that living with Danny and me might bring – the scratches and the screams and the head-banging at all hours of day or night – but they had also witnessed the pleasures, the heart-warming, subtle and unusual gifts and insights that come from knowing Danny, with his ability to experience joy and to share it exuberantly.

We started looking for a house that, if we pooled our resources, could accommodate us all – Adrian, Jamie, Josh, Danny, Corey and me. It had to be within the borders of Islington, because I knew how hard it can be to transfer support packages from one local authority to another. Danny's GP, his social worker, his personal budget, you name it – all these aspects of support would have to be reassessed, reappraised, very possibly changed and reduced, were we to leave our borough. So we were bound to Islington, and Adrian, Jamie and Josh had no choice but to make the move from Enfield, where they had been based. We found somewhere near to Finsbury Park station, an easy Tube ride back to Tami, the boys' mother, so that they could share their time between both parental homes.

By March 2011 we were settled in our new house, just around the corner from and similar to the previous one, but with the necessary additional bedrooms.

★

But the shadows didn't go away. Not only was Ingrid's absence a continuous presence, but more sadness was coming down the tracks. Donna and Paul's Daniel had been diagnosed with leukaemia. They were told that his chances were fifty–fifty.

By then Paul and Daniel were living in Suffolk. Paul did not leave Daniel's side in hospital through months of gruelling chemotherapy. Being over sixteen, Dan was assigned to an adult ward, even though he needed constant care and supervision, so Paul had to spend his nights as well as his days in a hospital chair.

During the spring of 2011, however, the leukaemia was officially in remission. At last they could go home for a while, even though daily chemo was still required. Paul was now learning how to administer this through lines in Dan's chest.

'Does the procedure worry you?' I asked him.

'No. The only thing I'm scared of these days is test results.'

Leukaemia underlined for Paul the conviction we had shared many years before regarding the vast difference between illness and autism. One conversation with Paul felt so important that I managed to write it down verbatim. This is what he said:

'Once you get to the core of it, it all becomes very straight-forward. I wouldn't change him for the world, and that's it. He still has his achievements, he still makes me laugh on a daily basis. And he's often a lot less trouble than his sister, who screams at me on a daily basis.' He chuckled.

'It's only the possible outcome that's a problem. I can deal with anything and everything else.'

But by August, Donna and Paul were required to face the unfaceable.

I received a text:

Hi Virginia, it's Paul – when you get a quiet moment could you give me a call for a chat?

So, while sitting outside in the midsummer sunshine, I phoned him.

'How's things?'

A pause. Then: 'Horrible horrible horrible' is his reply.

The disease has returned. Even the most aggressive treatment offers only a tiny percentage chance of survival.

Corey passes me some tissues as Paul and I talk and cry.

Daniel died on 12 September 2011.

I imagined the observations from more distanced folk. The platitudes about Paul being able at last to get on with his life, being able to devote himself entirely to the girls, being freed from the worry that some of us parents will have as our disabled children become adults and face the black hole that is the future without protective parental love.

And I wanted to punch these imagined commentators, repeatedly and forcefully, for their crass, ignorant comments. I extended this rage to those philosophers who have commented on disability and who don't know what they're talking about.

★

You'd think there might have been a chance for Daniel's family to have a bit of time, to withdraw from the world, to grieve, to stop struggling, to come to terms with the past and the gravity of their loss, without the interference of 'the system'.

But no.

Instead? What confronted them was Kafkaesque stupid stuff.

The death certificate needed the signature of two doctors, but the local Suffolk GP had never even met Daniel.

'Why didn't you ever introduce me to him?' the GP asked.

'He was under the hospital,' Donna replied. 'We didn't need you until he died.'

There ensued a protracted and farcical tour round East Anglia in the funeral director's car, chasing doctors, trying to find two who had known him.

Then Paul had to surrender the Motability car almost immediately, because Daniel's Disability Living Allowance was cut off instantly. No leeway to soften the blow, bearing in mind that Paul's whole life had been given over to supporting his son; he had neither time nor emotional capacity to get on his bike and job-search within a matter of days of Daniel's death.

And worst of all, Daniel's death didn't stop a punitive and vindictive court case against Donna and Paul. The allegation, which had already required two court hearings, was that the family had previously and fraudulently used Donna's council flat as a London base for Paul and Daniel, rather than for Donna, in whose name the flat was rented. Islington's fraud department pursued the case relentlessly, despite the fact that it was Donna herself who had innocently and in good faith brought the arrangement to their attention, along with her intention to resume occupancy of the flat.

Hugh – father of Jack and Ben – had acted as their dedicated housing lawyer through a series of complex interpretations of both housing law and family law. Now yet another hearing was scheduled, a retrial following the overturning of a previous judgment. It looked as though Donna and Paul were going to have to return to the witness stand and explain once again the decisions by which they had tried to support all their children when their needs were so different. To keep Daniel at TreeHouse, to enable the girls to thrive, to prevent Donna from sinking – all these themes would have been relived in court, under cross-examination, within weeks following Daniel's death, if the local authority lawyers had their way.

The welfare state was established, surely, so that we are less vulnerable to the vagaries of random, unbidden misfortunes. But sadly, it is also capable of abuse, towards the very people it is supposed to protect. The only thing that stopped this vindictive insensitivity and waste of local authority money and time was another piece of what you might call luck – though it's hard to use that word for such a dismal chain of events. An eleventh-hour reprieve, and a compromise was reached, whereby Donna agreed to move out of her flat and apply for a smaller one. Negotiations went to the wire, and only took place because I had once known the man who had recently taken up a senior post in the housing department. This smoothed the way to my approaching him directly. These connections – both with the senior housing person, and with Hugh, who gave everything to this case even though he was himself battling with ill health – were probably what stopped the retrial.

It shouldn't have to be like this.

34

HOME AND AWAY

During the autumn of 2011 it felt as if I were living in three different worlds.

In one, I was driven to distraction by what was happening to Donna and Paul, combining vicarious grief and outrage. The countdown to their court hearing involved a frenzy of negotiations and emails in which I was just one link in a long chain.

In my home, in contrast, the six of us were all acclimatising to one another well, in a chaotic but satisfactory arrangement in which our various carers, friends, partners all came and went with equal amounts of adaptability and goodwill. The difficult times didn't vanish, but Adrian, Jamie and Josh never complained about the constraints and challenges that Danny's periodic distress placed on them, and Danny reacted well to having three more men in his home.

One morning, a 5 a.m. knock on the bedroom door woke Adrian and me.

'Hello?'

'I don't mind,' were Jamie's first reassuring words, 'but I thought I should let you know: Danny came into my room, tapped my shoulder, got into bed with me, and has fallen asleep.'

It seemed important for Danny to learn that brotherly love requires alternative expression, so I guided him back to his room. But I was glowing with disbelieving gratitude. We really were a family now, and Danny was showing how much he welcomed this development.

And Josh, too. Younger than Jamie, he could have been forgiven for seeing Danny as more of a threat, or an embarrassment, but his loyalty has never, ever cracked. He was gentle and unfazed when a friend of his visited for the first time and Danny appeared naked. And he reacted with fury when his college tutor referred to someone in the class as a 'retard'. When challenged to explain what the tutor judged to be his overreaction, Josh said, 'My stepbrother has a learning disability. You should never talk like that about anyone.'

From Danny's expressions of joy on the garden swing, as from his episodes of pain and self-injury, the brothers learned quickly the profound intensity of Danny's humanity.

'He's the happiest and the saddest person I've ever met,' Jamie told Adrian.

In saying this, he touched upon one of the central themes of my later writing: how are we to judge what constitutes a good human life? On what criteria do we base our notions of well-being, happiness, attainment? What counts for more: a middle way (the middle of the bell curve, which might be deemed 'mediocrity'[1]) or the way of the outliers, whose existence might be more unusual, more extreme?

'When my daughter struggles, she does so considerably, however when she flies, she soars.'[2] These were the words of Helen Keeler, during her campaign to publicise the way she had been rejected as an egg donor because of her Asperger's daughter. She had then added this important reflection: 'I wonder if it is either possible or desirable to breed out these extreme states from our species.'

Helen was in effect asking precisely the research question I was posing. Is it right to try to prevent (conditions like)

autism? Further, is it right to deny potential parents the right
to choose?

So the lived experiences of Danny's and my home life, and
the insights that our now expanded family brought to us, flowed
right back into the broader issues of my research. And herein
lies the third of the worlds I inhabited in autumn 2011: when I
wasn't enjoying my family, and when I wasn't trying to support
Donna and Paul, my head was full of questions about the scientific and ethical issues that my thesis was tackling.

★

The ethical, legal and social implications (ELSI) of autism in
research were addressed in two USA-based workshops during
the autumn of 2011. I watched the proceedings of the first from
my home. Participants spoke and made recommendations that
were familiar territory to me. For example, the need for greater
dialogue among academics, families, autistic people, and the
need to shift the balance of autism research funding from cause
to interventions.[3]

The second workshop was to me altogether more significant
and novel. This was not just because it was hosted by the Autism
Self Advocacy Network (ASAN)[4] and half of its speakers were
autistic, but also because I was able to attend in person. What
extraordinary good fortune was this, to be sitting in Harvard
Law School and to see and hear firsthand the notable contributions of the speakers! It would never have dawned on me to try
to attend in person but for the suggestion of my doctoral supervisor, Mike Parker, who was able to access funding to make my
trip possible.

Another reason why I felt so lucky to be there is the fact that
I got to meet some of the people at the workshop – not just the
speakers but the rank-and-file members of ASAN, and other
autistic individuals who were interested enough to come along.

First, there was Ari Ne'eman, the founder of ASAN and the chair of the conference. Ari's CV is impressive: in 2009 he was the first autistic member of the US National Council on Disability and chair of its Policy and Program Evaluation Committee. He has authored an important book about the history of the disability rights struggle in the USA.[5]

He was a skilled and humorous chair of the workshop and gave me a warm greeting, based on a small amount of prior correspondence: 'Virginia, do you hug?'

I have learned to use this phrase with others, autistic and neurotypical alike, in moments when one should not assume how comfortable or uncomfortable another person might be with tactile greetings.

Another thing I took away and treasured was Ari's willingness, after the day's events and when no doubt exhausted, to sit together in the hotel lobby while he waited for a cab, and to respond patiently to my barrage of questions. He was kind and articulate, patient and friendly. His social stamina exceeded my own, which probably isn't what the old textbooks would have predicted.

But foremost among all of this was my good fortune in meeting a number of the people in the audience, the ASAN members who were there to listen rather than to speak. Some of us went for a drink afterwards – they invited me and I was on cloud nine. I expect I was a curiosity, a middle-aged Brit who'd come all the way from England even though the proceedings were going to be made available later on the internet. They were eager to tell me their stories. A troubled young man who was deeply alienated within his family, a warm and funny woman who teased me, a brainy scientist who had a biochemical theory about autism that was way beyond me, and so on.

At my next supervision, Mike asked me how the conference went.

'Oh it was great,' I enthused. 'I met some wonderful people.'

Just for a moment I think I saw a flash of consternation cross his face. I had to remember his point of view – that he didn't source the funds for me simply so that I could go out drinking with some nice folk in Boston. I gathered myself, and then outlined many of the things I learned from the speeches, and explained how valuable they would prove to be for my thesis.

Above all, what I took back was a greater understanding of the ways in which the scientific community, for all its emphasis on objectivity, can be unconsciously biased. Scientific data – which is supposedly beyond subjectivity – may actually be as open to interpretation as anything else. And in autism research, the deep error has been to assume that anything that is not 'normal' is by definition wrong, inferior, rather than just different, or even superior. Take, for example, some research I first heard about at the workshop.

The study had looked at how people behave in their charitable giving, according to whether or not they were being observed at the time of making a donation.[6] Neurotypicals varied their levels of generosity according to whether or not they were being watched. Seemingly keen to be regarded as generous, their donations increased when observed. Autistics, in contrast, gave consistently, with or without an audience. So the conclusion I would draw is that autistics are less preoccupied with what others will think of them than are NTs. But the researchers were more interested in the alleged 'inappropriateness' of the autistic behaviour. Unconscious bias towards NT behaviour occluded the researchers' ability to identify something valuable in how the autistics had behaved. There was no recognition that susceptibility to what others might think could be a sign of weakness and potential hypocrisy.

Another example in a similar vein is a study about the impact of oxytocin spray as a potential therapy for autistic people. The study found that oxytocin induced 'more appropriate social behaviour and affect'.[7] But what was this allegedly 'appropriate' behaviour? Having scrutinised the study, Michelle Dawson reached a very different conclusion. With characteristic humour, she identified and ridiculed the researchers' bias by pointing out that, actually, the autistics merely became greedier and more competitive in order to win:

> They learned and displayed selfishness and hypocrisy and us–vs–them thinking. Their objectivity, fairness, and altruism were – temporarily – cured.[8]

35

Surgery

The regime of daily flushes through the tube in Danny's side, which had seemed so promising back in 2010, started to fail after a year. By summer 2012, Danny's pain and violence levels seemed to escalate exponentially; he had an episode of dramatic bleeding from his rectum and thereafter his tube site was constantly leaking blood and faeces. We made repeated trips to A&E, having been bounced around various consultants who seemed reluctant to do much.

But suddenly everything changed. We finally had a long-promised appointment with Professor Knowles, consultant surgeon at the Royal London Hospital. Within five minutes of seeing Danny and hearing from me, he said: 'We've reached the end of the road. His bowel isn't working, the tube isn't functioning, and it's obviously urgent.'

Danny needed to undergo surgery to create a stoma, whereby his faeces would flow from an opening in the side of his abdomen into an external bag. This ileostomy, Professor Knowles's letter said, was 'the least destructive and safest measure that is best guaranteed to rectify the problem'.

Finally a doctor was saying the things that, deep down, I knew to be true. Danny should have a bag. No more enemas.

No more flushes through a tube that had stopped working. No more oozing of blood and excrement down his side. And – please oh please – no more pain?

Corey and I stayed with Danny in Intensive Care on the night after the surgery. The room seemed vast, excessively lit, full of murmurs and bleeps and the quiet thrumming of machinery. I lay beside Danny, having abandoned my mattress on the floor, in answer to his gesture for me to join him in his bed to hold him. Behind us, Corey lay on a second mattress, with us once again to face this latest challenge together. The nurse was serene and accommodating about this arrangement, and kept vigil over us with extraordinary calm. She really was called Angel.

I slept fitfully. I dreamt I was telling Ingrid all that had been happening. When I woke, I wished so much that I could see her and talk to her. And then immediately I was overcome with a huge weary certainty about my life. I wanted to stop doing all the things I had been doing in the wider world for over a decade. I had no energy or desire left to go to the meetings, to read the policy documents, to engage in the politics of disability and the autism movement. I was done in. It was a transient certainty, but at that point I started to feel a slow undertow of yearning – to write about the people in this book, to tell of the loves and connections that joined us in humanity. From then on, each time I was on the verge of being drawn into the fray more intensively, taking small tentative steps towards exploring job possibilities, or engaging in a new project, something would snap inside, as if I'd been stretching on an elastic tether as far as I could, only to find it pulling me back into a place of solitude and reflection.

Our stay in hospital didn't go smoothly. Although the operation seemed to go well, and Danny didn't seem too fazed by the ileostomy bag, he started post-operative projectile vomiting on the second day, and continued to do so for over a week.

The professor was on holiday, and at first the more junior doctors thought that Danny's vomiting was just a reaction to the anaesthetic. As the days wore on, and no amount of anti-emetic medication seemed to help, my worry started to build. Would his gut ever get its act together? Would he ever be able to eat his beloved crisps again? When Professor Knowles returned, he examined the charts, listened to our description of the symptoms, and said simply, 'Ileus. He's in ileus.' (Paralytic ileus – as it used to be termed when I was a junior nurse – is when the intestine goes on strike and is unable to pulsate and project its contents onwards.)

Finally, Danny's small intestine started to work again. But the experience of ten days of this massive 'overreaction' to surgery revealed a new feature of Danny's problems. A referral letter from Professor Knowles to his specialist colleague said:

All his situations are complicated by the autism, but *what we now know* also is that he has profound small bowel dysmotility and went into horrendous ileus after surgery. He has recently been treated for bacterial overgrowth for a worsening of his symptoms of pain ... [my italics]

What we now know.

What we now know.

Both reassuring and devastating.

We know more about why Danny has had pain for so long. That's good.

But we know too that the whole of his intestinal tract is compromised, and vulnerable to the twin challenges of bacterial build-up and a propensity to shut down – both of which cause dreadful pain. Not good.

I tucked my copy of this letter into my Filofax and for several years carried it with me. What we now know.

No more 'Am I making too much fuss?' Instead, the need for vigilance in monitoring all his symptoms, adjusting the medication and pain relief, restricting his diet drastically. And an even greater need to relish the times when he is well and cheerful, when his exuberance and humour return, when he jumps for joy on a windy day, or smiles to hear the Beatles, and shouts with glee on the swing.

★

Danny didn't take long to get accustomed to having a stoma bag. After a few dramatic occasions when he experimented with removing it, he soon settled. The need for a mass clear-up and shower (he hates showers), and the interruption while bedsheets were changed, proved an effective disincentive to further tampering with the bag – although of course accidents will always happen. In any case, I found these early episodes of mayhem reassuringly straightforward, because they proved I had been right in my assertion to the medics pre-operatively that 'I would rather clear away a houseful of shit than have Danny go through this much pain.'

There was a short period of gung-ho confidence, and then we were back in the land of torment again. Professor Knowles's referral to his colleague presaged a journey of discovery in which we would gradually unravel the layers of challenges that Danny faced. We would be referred to new doctors in neurology (for input on pain management), allergy and immunology (for an insight into the nature of, and how best to respond to, his altered immune state) and rheumatology (which confirmed a condition of hypermobility). They would all shed light on a condition of the connective tissue (Ehlers–Danlos syndrome, or EDS), with which autism may – or may not – be intimately connected.[1]

This journey had a direct parallel in the thesis I was writing. I was convinced that all Danny's suffering was linked to his medical problems, rather than to his autism or learning disability. I also noticed that many who espoused treatment for autism were actually often referring to 'add-ons' – epilepsy, gut problems, anxiety – conditions that didn't fall within the core symptoms that confer a diagnosis of autism. When calling for treatment, or cure, they were really calling for treatment for additional conditions that some – but not all – autistic people experience. And, I might add, these were also conditions that some – but not all – neurotypical people experience.

This difference between the core condition and susceptibility to other conditions is so important that it justifies further analogies to drive home the point: if ovarian cancer is a problem to be treated, you do just that. What you do not do is pathologise all women. And in heritable conditions such as sickle-cell, it is sensible to seek out susceptibility where a causative agent is known, rather than eliminating an entire ethnic group on account of their particular vulnerability.[2]

I have used this argument in my doctoral research, in my writing and in public forums.[3] And over the years I have noticed that these ideas are gaining some traction. A contemporary multi-site consortium uses the language of 'comorbidities' to justify genetic research, rather than talking about treatment or cure of autism itself.[4]

So if the spotlight is on the conditions to which autistic people are particularly susceptible, but not on their core autistic and/or learning-disabled being, does that clear a way for genetic research to progress full steam ahead?

I still have some nagging worries about all of this. My concern is twofold.

First, it is possible that some of the comorbidities are triggered by social/environmental conditions, rather than by the biochemistry of the autistic person. Take depression and anxiety, for example. A recent study found a strong link between the quality of life of autistic people and the incidence of these mental health problems.[5] Research has also found a correlation between suicidality and the degree to which autistic people have felt impelled to disguise or hide their autism.[6] If autistic people did not feel so stigmatised, bullied, excluded, might this not reduce their levels of depression and anxiety, which in turn would improve their quality of life? Do we need to look at their genes, or do we need to look at the social attitudes that undermine their self-esteem, access to employment or a sense of belonging? Or, if we are looking at genes, and pouring millions of pounds into the research effort, should we not at least pour an equal amount of money into anti-bullying campaigns, broader anti-discrimination initiatives and appropriate skills training for teachers, social workers, employers? An autistic person's melt-downs will be prevented or handled far more effectively by a skilled and empathetic practitioner who has been trained, supervised and rewarded appropriately, than by an untrained, unsupervised, low-paid and undervalued member of staff (which is what happens far too often in the current social care system).

My second concern relates to the list of comorbidities that are lumped together as medical issues. In the current diagnostic criteria, learning disability and challenging behaviour are ranged alongside epilepsy and gastrointestinal problems. But only the latter are potentially fatal, organic illnesses that are independent of external conditions, and therefore I consider epilepsy and gastrointestinal problems to be conceptually distinct from other areas in which some autistic people experience difficulties.

I was thinking a lot about this in the autumn of 2012, when the dual preoccupation of my ethics research and Danny's illness came to a head, and I wrote the following in my journal.

30 November 2012

I am imagining a future world in which prospective mothers, thanks to pre-implantation genetic diagnosis, will be

forearmed with information that their future child will have
a debilitating gut problem along with autism and learning
disability. That the autism and learning disability may render
him charming, adorable, wonderful and capable of great joy,
but that the gut problem will blight his life, bring on violence
and make those around him frightened of him – from time
to time.

*If I had been told this before Danny was born, what would
I have done?*

Would I have been cruel to continue with the pregnancy
in the knowledge of future pain, or would I have been right
to emphasise the profound compensation, for him and those
around him, brought by all the joy and pleasure he would
experience and bring to others?

I am so very glad I did not have this information when I was
pregnant, and did not have to make a choice.

36

Spring and Summer 2013

It seems I was in a period of intense introspection during these months, judging by the frequency of my journal entries. Some of what I wrote is as follows.

15 May 2013

An envelope from the DWP (Dept. for Work and Pensions) contains some excellent news. They have looked again at Danny's Disability Living Allowance and now confirm that his entitlements are indefinite. Thank the Lord. It means that aspect of Danny's future relationship with the welfare state is settled (at least, until some potential future government moves the goalposts again).

Strange looking back at school, and Oxford, and the 'glittering prizes' that were held out in those days. Strange contemplating the extraordinary success of some of my contemporaries. I was never going to be one of them, the OBE notwithstanding. Despite bonkers things like the press conference with Arsène Wenger and the visits to Downing Street or TV studios,[1] I am basically the woman who sits here in the kitchen, having slept off the effects of three consecutive nights of small-hours stoma-bag changes for Danny, privately celebrating a letter from the DWP.

20 May 2013

All the time, *all the time*, I seem to be trying to wrestle with how we shore up a benevolent welfare state and cradle the vulnerable as if they were our own family. The vulnerable we always carry with us. We *are* the vulnerable, all of us, at some stage during our lives, and particularly as we decline, fade and die. And if not us, then our children and grandchildren, and if not them, then the families of people who clean our offices, process our sewage, grow our food. The people we brush past in the streets, the people we inadvertently cause to suffer thousands of miles away as a result of adverse trade conditions, tax evasion, weapons manufacture and sales. We are all in this together. We all affect one another. John Donne.

6 June 2013

When Danny was in his bath, he was happier and more joyful than any other nineteen-year-old you could possibly imagine. When he got out of the bath and let me wrap him in the towel, he laughed and chuckled in his unique Danny way, and I caught the thought in me, clear and certain: 'Of all the possible other children I could have had, you are preferred to all of them.'

I had been reflecting on the issue of 'procreative benefi- cence', whereby, according to some philosophers, we are morally obliged to choose, of all potential children, the one

who will have the best chance of the best life.[2] These philosophers say that on the balance of probabilities and available
data, being disabled predicts a lower quality of life than not
being disabled. So one should not choose, if one has alternatives, the potentially disabled embryo.

But how can we know, really, of all our potential children,
who will have the best chance of the best life, or even a
decent chance of a good life? Of all the other possible children who might have emerged, I want only Danny. So what
do they know, really, about what's important, and what
makes us who we are?

19 July 2013

Danny and I both awake since 3 a.m. He is now, at 7.30 a.m.,
out on the hammock, swinging and smiling and watching
the trees gently swaying and saying 'oyee, ah-ee' from time
to time in total contentment.

And so began Danny's final year at TreeHouse. Rather wonderful for its lack of drama, it entailed a remarkably easy process of
Person-Centred Planning in relation to his next placement.[3]
The journey from children's to adult services is often tortuous
and frightening. Young people and their families have to engage
with new personnel, new benefits entitlements, new hurdles to
identify the right move post-school. They then face the possibility that there will again be differences of opinion about this,
and the usual argument about funding.

But once again we were luckier than many. We were
supported by a stellar team of Belinda Blank at TreeHouse and
Beth Cox at London Borough of Islington, both of whom
were employed specifically to facilitate transitions such as
Danny's, and they helped us every step of the way. By then

TreeHouse's new chief executive, Jolanta Lasota, and her dynamic colleague Andy Lusk, were setting up a unique post-school service that would combine the best of college-based education and home-based support.

So it was agreed and sorted. Danny would attend a new scheme based at Barnet College but run by the TreeHouse charity. That way he could continue to benefit from its educational approach – including ABA – with which he was familiar and comfortable. After he had spent so many years at the school, I knew it wouldn't be easy for Danny, going to a new building and meeting new tutors, and I knew too that on the first day I would feel as raw as I had all those years ago when I left him with his new childminder. But still, I felt as confident as one could be that when the time came for Danny to leave TreeHouse school – in the summer of 2013 – he would be assured a safe and stable passage.

37

CRISIS

Back in 2002, I was overwhelmed by the story of Helen Rogan, who killed herself and her autistic son Mark Owen because successive cries for help and more support came to nothing. The isolation and exhaustion eroded her energy and hope, and became deadly and murderous.

Year after year, there are similar tales. It is sometimes whispered in dark corners, and sometimes said more openly, that parents fantasise about a simultaneous death for them and their disabled child. And it is said more loudly, and more frequently, that parents of disabled children often hope that they can outlive their child. Experience has taught them that much of the social care system is on its knees, that any semblance of adequate support relies on parents being forever alert. Who will take up the battle when they are gone?[1]

I cannot avoid this, when telling you what happened in the late summer of 2013.

I am wearing my scarlet dressing gown, made of towelling material, decorated with a yellow Arsenal logo. My faithful dressing gown, beloved by me, given by my mother as a Christmas present some years back. If you were to spot me — on CCTV, say, or from the far end of a corridor — you would see a lone figure, pacing up and down in the darkness, restlessly and distractedly wringing her hands, the bright red of the dressing gown incongruous against the colourless gloom of the surroundings. All is quiet save for the whirring of the distant hospital generator, the beeps of monitors and the occasional footsteps of nursing staff as they work the night shift while their patients sleep.

I am pacing and hand-wringing like a demented person in bright red, realising what a strange figure I must present, but beyond all ability to compose my thoughts or contain my movements of distress.

Monday

Danny had been taken to hospital in an ambulance in the small hours. Adrian and I had accompanied him, and stayed with him in A&E as various personnel came and went between 2 and 6 a.m. Danny was by then calm and sleepy, having been given maximum pain relief in the previous hours at home, waiting for the paramedics. By 6 a.m., still behind the curtains in our A&E cubicle, Adrian and I are fighting sleep, and wondering if this is all some kind of overreaction on our part. Then finally the relevant doctor arrives, takes one look at Danny's bulbous stoma, which looks like a swollen beetroot rather than the little red strawberry of its healthy days, and explains to us that they are getting the operating theatre ready for emergency surgery that will shortly be started by the general surgical team. The procedure cannot wait until the arrival of the colorectal surgeons under whose specialty Danny resides. And in any case, the surgeon who knows Danny best – Professor Knowles – is away.

This is not, to say the least, what we have been expecting. While appreciating its seriousness – otherwise why call for an ambulance at 1 a.m.? – I have not considered the possibility that

Danny's situation is so critical that even a further hour without intervention could be disastrous.

Everything swings into action. We are suddenly all motion as his trolley is wheeled to another anonymous bay, and then another. While forms are signed and identity checked and rechecked, I am saying to Adrian, 'I don't believe this.' I cannot believe that after a year of such progress, and – at long last – of *hope*, we are back, seemingly, to square one, or worse: square zero, square minus-one.

At 7 a.m. we phone Nick. Amanda answers the phone and I ask straightaway for Nick, saying that Danny is in hospital again. When he comes to the phone he immediately asks, 'What chance does he have if things have got this bad so quickly, and after he was doing so well?' I don't remember what answer I gave. When I phone Corey he says he's on his way before I've even finished the sentence.

Nick and Corey both arrive at the hospital as soon as they can, but by then the operation has started. Adrian and I have been there in the anaesthetic room, I to sing to Danny and stroke him as he gazes into my eyes, and Adrian helping to restrain him from fighting the needle and the descent into unconsciousness.

It is that strange limbo time, while Danny is under and the medics are doing what needs to be done, and the four of us hover above the City on a glass bridge that joins two tower blocks. Outside it is bright and sunny, the sky is a cheery blue and the tall buildings gleam. Finally Adrian leaves, with tears in his eyes, amidst hugs for us all, and Corey walks with him to the exit for a smoke.

So there are two of us – Nick and me – on the glass bridge hovering over the City. The air conditioning is fierce, and we shiver. Nick tells me that he has a big decision to make. He has just been given a tight deadline to make substantial adjustments to a film script for Reese Witherspoon. Filming has already started, so no delay is possible. Either he should hand it over to someone else, now, or he should press on and do the rewrite himself – but will as a result be less available to support Danny during working hours over the coming days.

'Do you have a view on what I should do?' he asks.

It seems obvious to me how the division of labour should fall. I do not mean it as a reproach, but the reality is this: Corey and I are old hands regarding Danny's hospitalisations, I say, and meanwhile it's in all our interests if we focus on what we do best – Nick should, if he can, press on with the film script.

Reese Witherspoon will later be nominated for an Oscar for her role in the film *Wild*, scripted by Nick. But at that time of its early shooting, and Nick's rapid rewrite of sections, I only know that she is sending Danny messages of support which Nick passes on. It is kind of her, and her fame, which might at another time have impressed or intimidated me, is now only something that adds to the sense of unreality about what is happening to us all.

While Danny is in the recovery area, still unconscious, the surgeon comes to talk to us. Danny has done well, he says, and all is in order again.

'There is a laparotomy wound, but we only had to remove a small section of his intestine, and we have managed to create a new stoma in the same place as the old one.' This is all, apparently, very good news.

'And what caused it?'

'It was an intussusception, a twisting of the intestine, which then cut off the blood supply and killed the section of the intestine that we had to remove.'

'What are the chances of this happening again in the future?' Nick asks.

'These things are very rare. Hopefully it will never happen again.' The surgeon then qualifies this, and says in technical terms what I translate into words that I can more confidently repeat: Danny's intestines are unusually floppy, so the risk is greater for him than for most people. But still, they have done something additional this time round, which makes the chance of a repetition less likely.

I am content to take everything at face value. There is no time to look into the longer term because we need to be at Danny's bedside as he recovers, checking he doesn't worry away at the wound and the new stoma, ensuring he doesn't pull out the drip, dealing with the frequent beeps as the monitor intermittently falters, and just being there to watch him drift in and out of sleep, stroking his hands, telling him we love him, overseeing the regular observations and drug administration undertaken by the nursing staff.

Monday passes in this fashion. Nick goes back to work. Corey and I stay and take it in turns to have breaks. I text college to explain that Danny won't be in, and I call my mother, to change the arrangements we had previously made for this day. Adrian sends lovely messages of love and support. The hours pass. The day passes. The night passes.

Tuesday

By Tuesday morning Danny should be a bit better, and as we face another day, Corey and I are reasonably sanguine. The nurse allocated to Danny for the day shift is an elderly Indian woman who used to be a ward manager and who still works part-time. Her experience, calm and skill fill us with confidence, and though we are tired, there seems to be a way forward on this new day.

But Danny is not any better. His respirations are far too rapid; he is, if anything, paler than before; and his blood pressure is falling dangerously low. The nurse's experience tells her that things aren't good, and we are thankful for her authority, which

probably hastens the speed of more doctor visitations, greater
frequency of monitoring and a hastily arranged trip down to
X-ray. Instead of waiting for a porter, which is taking forever, she
and Corey set off together, pushing Danny's trolley on their own.

I take the opportunity of their absence from the ward to lie
down on the mattress on the floor, and fall asleep. Within
minutes a man I don't recognise comes into the room, and I
peer up at him sleepily. He seems disconcerted to find me in
such a state. I stand up, composing myself as quickly as I can to
hear the news: Danny is bleeding inside. He needs to go back to
the operating theatre immediately. The doctor has already
signed the consent form because 'in situations like this you only
need a doctor's signature'.

His phone rings and he answers it. From his tone and from
his responses, I gather that a colleague on the surgical team is
calling him.

'Yes, I've seen them,' he says (which I translate as: yes, I've
seen the X-rays of Danny's abdomen).

'*Shit*, man!' I hear the person at the other end of the phone
exclaim. So loud and emphatic is his delivery that his words are
audible to anyone nearby, and there's no mistaking the fact that
Danny is in big trouble.

'Er, I'm with his mother now,' the surgeon says quickly, clearly
aware that his colleague's turn of phrase was not intended for
anyone else's ears.

And then Danny returns from the tell-tale X-ray, deathly
white, mute and immobile on his bed, which is pushed by
Corey and the nurse. Immediately there are people rushing
around, putting up bags of blood – which are in turn surrounded
by pressure cuffs to hasten the pace of the transfusions. And
then we're off again, our little group, back towards the anaesthetic room, to more singing and stroking and loving words for
Danny as he is drugged into unconsciousness for the second
time in two days, and his abdomen is once again opened up.

The only memory I have of the period of Danny's second operation is a text I send to my sister Jane. 'Danny back in theatre for haemorrhage. I can hardly bear it, but have to.'

John comes in to cover the night shift with me, even though he's been working all day and will be again tomorrow. He is angry with fate for letting Danny down so badly and I appreciate what this says about how much he cares. For my own part I can feel no anger, but I'm very grateful for John's.

Wednesday morning

Nick, Adrian, Corey and I have convened at Danny's bedside. This time, Danny has three drains from his abdomen in addition to the original one, and a urinary catheter as well as the drips into his arms, along with the dressing on the – now longer – abdominal wound and a bag over the newly refashioned stoma.

Corey is urging us to ask for a special nurse to be allocated to Danny, because we are getting to the point of exhaustion and Danny cannot be left alone. I'm still wearing the clothes I was wearing on Sunday. A plan is hatched. Adrian will bring in supplies of clothes, toiletries, books and treats; we will start texting round his wider circle of carers – not just Sarah and John but also his tutors from college – and ask them to come in and do a shift or two; and we will talk to the ward manager about whether they can obtain some extra agency-nurse support.

Nick and I go outside for a smoke. He is as broken as I've ever seen him. He is wretched about the latest turn of events, he is wretched about feeling he's abandoned Danny in order to finish a script – notwithstanding that I encouraged this – and he is wretched about Danny's prospects. I tell him that he's a wonderful father, and that Danny is not going to die, that side-effects and mishaps are sadly routine but that Danny will pull through just fine.

Wednesday afternoon

In the afternoon Sarah comes in. She has rallied to the call, she has taken an afternoon off work and here she is at Danny's bedside, with the up-to-date knowledge of monitoring equipment from her recent children's nursing work that I do not possess. What Sarah notices is that Danny's oxygen saturation readings on the monitor are dangerously low.

If it weren't for Sarah, we would have let valuable hours slip by without alerting anyone to this new danger. Thanks to her, time is saved, so that by the time her stint has finished and she is handing over to David – Danny's ABA supervisor – doctors are requiring regular arterial blood samples to be taken from Danny, and organising an emergency set of tests and a chest X-ray.

Despite his depleted state and limited consciousness, Danny's instinct is still to pull away firmly from an approaching needle; it needs a man's strength to hold his arm firm to prevent injury while the arterial blood samples are taken, and so David's arrival is well-timed. During his stint supporting Danny over the next couple of hours, David will act as porter/bed-pusher, nurse and moral support, all with calm and kindness. Once again, protocols are shunted aside: this time it is David, me and two doctors who wheel Danny's bed down corridors and in and out of lifts in order to have yet another emergency X-ray.

By now Danny has an oxygen mask and we are under strict instructions not to let the reading on the monitor fall below ninety-five. A specialist nurse called Abi is also involved. She seems to carry as much authority and decision-making power as the medical staff. She explains to us that both Danny's lungs have partially collapsed.

Now Abi is making a treatment plan for Danny. She wants urine samples taken from the catheter at regular intervals; she will insert a nasogastric tube through Danny's nostril into his stomach to prevent vomiting; and she is also warning about the possibility of chest drains. I have lost count of all the tubes and drains conveying substances into Danny's body, and draining away others. His output is variously blood red, shit brown, bilious green and urinary gold, while the fluids and oxygen entering him are discreetly neutral in colour.

I am told that the lungs should gradually restore their shape, at which point his blood oxygen reading will reach the magic level of ninety-five without the need for oxygen to be administered. In the meantime, a permanent vigil is required to ensure he doesn't pull off the mask which enables the oxygen levels to hold up, or – if he does push it to one side – to intervene immediately to put it back in position.

Wednesday evening

Because of the need for such constant attention, and such a large entourage, Danny has now been moved to a big room of his own, and there is a proper bed for his overnight carer, as well as ample space for multiple nursing and medical staff should they be necessary.

But for a while I am alone with Danny, letting everything sink in. Soon I am joined by the surgeon who on the previous day had conveyed the news that Danny needed a second emergency operation. This time he is here to tell me that all is now well with the abdomen, but that it is vitally important that Danny mobilises in order to prevent further lung complications.

I baulk at this. How is Danny to mobilise when he is so weak, recovering from surgery on consecutive days, when he is moreover encumbered by drips, drains, catheters and an oxygen mask, and when in any case his severe learning disability means that he will not understand what is required, or why, and is therefore unlikely to cooperate?

'I don't care if he pulls all his drains out,' the surgeon almost barks, seemingly irritated. 'He must mobilise.' End of. He leaves.

On several occasions, friends and I have talked about why some surgeons do not possess greater communication skills. We have argued that perhaps this is an inevitability. For someone to have the nerve, courage and skill to cut people open and make life-saving decisions, and perform procedures requiring extraordinary focus and calm, they may in turn have to eschew traits of self-doubt and sensitivity that would encumber such vital work – even if in so doing they come over as arrogant or brash to their patients and their patients' families.

So I do not begrudge him his lack of communication skills on this occasion.

Unfortunately, though, the tone and content of his message leave me poleaxed. It feels to me that he is asking for the inhumane as well as the impossible, and at the same time telling me that only such inhumane and impossible actions will save Danny's life, and moreover that in expressing my doubts I am being obstructive.

And so it is that I am found weeping by a new nurse on duty and an agency nurse who has been assigned to 'special' Danny for the night.

If I hadn't been found weeping, would things have been different?

On the one hand, the nurses would have found me as I was: a tired, worried mother, who had had three days of bad and then worsening news, back to back, about her beloved son, who was now critically ill. A mother who had been with him virtually the whole time, and who had had very little sleep. Of course I was weeping, of course I was bewildered by what the surgeon had been telling me. Of course it was all too much.

On the other hand, perhaps empathy clouded their sense of what needed to be done overnight. Perhaps in their sympathy they judged wrongly that my need for untroubled sleep was greater than Danny's need for vigilance.

Whatever the reason, an error of judgement was about to take place that would plunge me and Danny into the deepest pit of all.

Wednesday night

The agency nurse encourages me to sleep. I have explained in detail what is needed, as has the nurse in charge. In no particular order: regular checks to abdominal wound; regular checks to urine output; regular checks to drains; regular checks of intravenous drip, nasogastric tube, stoma bag. And above all: permanent focus on the oxygen mask, so that if he brushes it aside, you put it back in place. Minute by minute, second by second, the oxygen mask needs to be in place.

I am urged to lie down on the bed that has now been made available, while the agency nurse sits at Danny's bedside watching over him carefully. I observe them both for a while, I see her gently adjust his oxygen mask at regular intervals, and I fall asleep.

Several hours later I am woken by sounds of rapid footsteps and urgent whispering. There is a small commotion around Danny's bed. I sit up, pull on my Arsenal dressing gown and walk over.

Danny is lying in, and is covered head to toe with, liquid faecal matter that has somehow leaked from the stoma bag. The oxygen mask is off. The reading on the monitor is eighty-five.

A nurse goes off to fetch clean linen, wet wipes, towels.

For the past three days, Danny has been virtually silent. We have not heard his familiar oy oy oys, nor even faint grunts. He hasn't made eye contact, as he is usually so fond of doing, and there have been no smiles. When not asleep, he has lain still, looking into the middle distance, and his breath has been shallow. We have continued to talk to him softly and stroke his hand and tell him how brilliantly he is doing, but he is not well enough to respond, though he remains cooperative when the nurses do their observations, when we wash him and change his sheets. But now, as he lies there, he seems further gone than ever. It's as if he's given up. He has not had the strength, it seems, to convey any kind of protest at lying in a pool of faeces. And his entire chemistry must be going awry in response to the drop in oxygen saturation.

In the few seconds that I watch, I imagine two nightmare scenarios simultaneously. One is a catastrophic infection – there can surely be no way the abdominal incision wound and the drain wounds can withstand the bacterial onslaught of the faecal matter that seems to be covering him. The other is acidosis caused by his low oxygen readings. This, I have inferred through what has not been said, can be disastrous. My poor poor darling Danny – what terrible thing has happened, to find you in such a state? And where was I while this was happening? I was so very near you but I was *asleep. I was not there to protect you.*

My instincts are to push the nurses to one side and to take over, though I realise that, whatever the neglect that has led to this state of affairs, they are at least more competent than I to do all that is necessary now – to clean him up swiftly, to restore the drips and drains and tubes to their rightful place, to make him comfortable again. And if I just stand and watch I am merely in the way, as well as being in danger of blurting out words and unintelligible noises that I will later regret.

So I leave the three of them, overwhelmed by how helpless I have become in the face of Danny's own helplessness and vulnerability. I go and pace the ward corridors in my dressing gown, trying not to scream, howl, wail and sob like some demented creature in the darkest hour of the night. I wring my hands, I clench and unclench them. I fall apart.

I cannot believe that this thing has happened to Danny.

I cannot believe that at the point when he faced his greatest danger and his greatest degradation, I was not there to look after him and protect him.

These facts are as near to being unbearable as anything will ever be again in my life.

The pain of this is followed by a moment of seeming clarity.

Danny is not safe without me, even for a short time while I am sleeping.

But I cannot survive without sleep.

The logical impossibility of squaring these propositions is evident. There is no way out.

And now I am approaching the place of predecessors whose tragedies have occasionally come to public attention. Helen Rogan and Mark Owen. Mothers whose passionate love and exhaustion and sense of their own indispensability lead them to commit terrible acts of violence to their children and themselves; a joint act of murder and suicide. The place from which such choices are made unites unendurable pain with a terrible logic, one that leads to a belief that two deaths are preferable to any possible alternative future.

When Danny is again clean and his oxygen mask is once more the focus of constant vigil, and when I have learned that the problem happened because the agency nurse hadn't wanted to wake me when she took her break (and I don't want to know how long that break was …) and the other nurses were too busy to stay with Danny all the time, I search for some paper and a writing implement. All I have is my sudoku book, so I scribble on one of its pages these words: *I will have to stay awake for the rest of my life.*

And then I realise that this may not be long enough. So I add: *And the rest of Danny's life.*

★

In the ensuing days, Danny did at last start to make progress. More reinforcements arrived to join the vigil on the ward, in the persons of Ben and Vincent (two of his college tutors), Lee, and Aine (Michele's daughter). All took turns, and together with Nick's daily visits, and the stints that Sarah and John offered on top of their day jobs, enabled Corey and me to have breaks to shower and sleep in a nearby Ibis hotel.

And finally Danny came home. We entered a hallowed place.

6 September 2013

Still he has this beatific smile. First thing in the morning, when I go in to see him lying in bed, he smiles up at me. This afternoon, after we both slept on his bed with my arm around him, he woke and started tapping at the iPad, then turned to me with that same angel smile.

He has a gaping wound in the centre of his lower abdomen that needs cleaning, packing and re-dressing every day by the district nurse. There is fresh blood and it occasionally mixes with the faeces in the bag stuck to the right side of his lower abdomen. And yet he behaves as if life has just given him the most amazing gift – the gift of simply being alive, of having fun, of a swing waiting for him out in the garden, and crisps waiting for him in the kitchen cupboard, and an army of people surrounding him with love.

I hear his sounds through the day as he interacts with his tutors, happy whoops and contented oy oy oys. It's as if life has got even better for him over the past few weeks. And as if those days in hospital took him into a place of wisdom or grace: some learning about what one can – and what one cannot – influence, what one has to accept because there is no alternative, and what one can thereby appreciate, because all that is above the non-negotiable is pure gift.

★

For nearly eight months, district nurses came daily to clean and re-dress the abdominal wound, which over-granulated and became infected, but did finally heal to leave an assertive but untroubling scar. Danny stoically endured early-morning starts to attend college part-time, and finally he was able to bathe again, go swimming, trampoline and regain his former life patterns.

Somehow Danny had escaped the worst scenarios I envisaged during that dark night of the soul, and he taught me that despite the seeming logic of my unhinged thoughts, the choices and the consequences were not mine to decide. They were down to him and the capacity for healing within him that no one else could gainsay. I could love him and advocate for him with all the resources my heart and brain could muster, but his strength and his stoicism and his sense of humour and his ability to inspire love were *his and his alone*, and I needed above all to respect and nurture those, and never impose my own despair on his hopeful and innocent soul, his inner core of strength. To lose hope and faith in his resilience would have been the greatest of sins.

And with that knowledge, that awareness of the firm boundary that exists between my love for Danny and his own, separate, will to live, I was ready to contemplate the next stage of our lives.

Within a year we were making plans for Danny to move to Leigh Road – a new Islington housing development for adults with learning disabilities, situated exactly halfway between Nick's house and mine, and providing individualised support according to the needs of each tenant. And the final chapters of my thesis were taking form. It was as if we were racing away as fast as we could from those terrible days in the Royal London Hospital.

Part 6

UNCERTAINTY AND BELIEF

'I have abandoned
my theories, the easier certainties
of belief.'

R. S. Thomas, 'Balance'

The events at the Royal London Hospital in the summer of 2013 were a watershed. I was forever changed. Since then I have recognised more fully than I had before that Danny is the resilient master of his own destiny and I must follow his lead, notwithstanding his need for vigilant care and unconditional love, and the possibility of more crises ahead that are beyond anyone's control. My job is to support him and the other people who are also supporting him, but not consider myself indispensable. I have to let him fly, as far as he is able, in the knowledge that one day I will not be there to protect him.

In a completely different way, summer 2013 was also seismic for the wider autism community. The diagnostic criteria for autism underwent a massive revision.

What follows addresses some of the burning questions that haven't gone away, stimulated as so often by the people we have met and the things they have taught us.

38

DISAGREEMENTS AND THE EMPATHY QUESTION

The idea that autistic people don't have the capacity for empathy, while neurotypicals do, is a familiar trope. It is used as a shorthand demarcation between autistic and non-autistic ways of being, thinking and feeling. The notion that autistic people have 'zero degrees of empathy' was outlined by Simon Baron-Cohen in his book of that name.[1] I should stress that he did distinguish between types of empathy: the type that is about relating to what others might be thinking (cognitive empathy) and the ability to care at a feeling level (affective empathy). While autistic people have limited cognitive empathy, he argued, they do have the capacity to care about other people.

But is it as simple as this? Are such demarcations accurate, and are they useful? Moving the debate onwards, Dr Damian Milton – whose experience of autism spans both his own (late-diagnosed) condition and that of his son – authored a seminal essay on 'double empathy'. He pointed out that problems between autistic people and NTs arise due to difficulties in *mutual* misunderstanding, and cannot be located solely within an autistic person.[2]

This was an important challenge to the simplistic idea that you can separate NTs from autistics on the basis of empathy.

Charming NTs can make others feel good, they can stroke other people's egos, they perhaps have an ability to know what will encourage the other person to like them, but they can still be callous. In other words, they have 'good social skills', which is something that may be very different from kindness or genuine concern.

And surely empathy is something that NTs are good at switching on and off – for example, when walking past beggars in the street.[3] In contrast, at least some autistic people seem to find it much harder to switch off. I came across the following passage from a blog:

> Understand I have too much empathy, I feel too much when I see others distress and pain, so I shut down sometimes.
>   When I want to confort [*sic*] you I normally don't know how, believe I am more worried for you than you can think.[4]

This highlights an important distinction between social skills (she doesn't know how to offer comfort) and the capacity for empathy (she actually feels 'too much').

I am not sure we have even begun to scratch the surface with regard to autism and empathy. I say this not just because of what has been written and debated about it, but also because of the people who have influenced me in recent years.

Ros

Ros Blackburn inspired Sigourney Weaver's portrayal of the autistic protagonist Linda Freeman in the film *Snow Cake*.[5]

My own encounters with Ros were always rewarding. She had been one of the first autistic people in the UK to speak publicly about her condition, and my first memory of her was at a conference soon after Danny's diagnosis in the late 1990s.

She talked about how autism affected her life, how it held her back, how it prevented her from acquiring certain skills and attributes (navigating trains, going to the shops), and how it made her dependent on her parents and terrified of a future without them. Her delivery was nonetheless cheerful and full of humour. On one occasion,[6] we were both panellists at a conference at which the complex ethical issues around cure and prevention were aired.

Years later we both spoke in a similar vein at another conference.[7] On my way home afterwards, I had a drink in the bar that overlooked the concourse at the railway station. A very loud group of young, drunk white men were behaving as though they had sole and unquestionable right to the space and to make their presence felt, regardless of the needs and preferences of other travellers. They were determined to cause discomfort, intent on drowning out the announcements on the tannoy. I thought back to the conference, attended by many autistics as well as NTs, and reflected how everyone had behaved with courtesy and consideration, unlike this puerile and boorish rabble here, who seemed devoid of any capacity for empathy with their fellow travellers.

I thought about Ros.

'Ros, you are a much, much finer person than any of this lot,' I wanted to say to her. 'It is an *injustice*, rather than a failing in you, that you have experienced so many problems and obstacles in your life, while they flaunt their arrogance with abandon.'

Chris and Sam

Chris and Sam are two young autistic friends of mine, and we meet in our local café from time to time. Sam is often depressed; he berates himself for his inability to thrive in the world as it is.

He longs to be free of his disability. In contrast, Chris, who is very protective of Sam, argues that in the case of their autism, society's failings are to blame for the problems they both have. He cites widespread obstruction and discrimination, and he wants to campaign to make the world a more accommodating place for everyone. They are the best of friends, and their different ways of viewing the world and themselves do not impede their relationship or tip them into the kind of hostile name-calling that often happens on social media.

I met Sam and Chris for one of our catch-ups in the local café recently. I asked them how it would be if I wrote about them, and they agreed to see a draft. I explained that between them they manifested the different views about autism as disability to be lamented vs autism as difference requiring accommodation.

Chris looked at Sam and said with a grin: 'I know what Sam's thinking.'

Ta-da!

Here was a spontaneous, real-life, 'from the horse's mouth' refutation of the notion that autistic people possess no 'cognitive empathy',[8] or theory of mind.[9] With one phrase, Chris overturned the oft-repeated certainty that autistic people struggle to imagine other people's mental states.

He continued: 'You're wondering if the book will turn into a film, aren't you, Sam?'

Sam – an avid filmgoer – agreed, and they were both amused, as was I. They went on to talk about the fact that they do disagree with one another quite often, but that it doesn't threaten their friendship. And in so doing they added another nail in the coffin of the assertion that autistic people cannot reflect on their own mental states or their own interactions.[10]

The truth is, they both struggle in our world, and cause minimal harm. And they face their challenges (for example, isolation, financial abuse, the time it takes for the DWP to respond) with friendliness, patience and deep courage. The unfairness of this situation burns through me. They have such admirable qualities, but not many people take the trouble to discover them. I think of the repellent people who inflict damage with their (often misplaced) 'I own the world' confidence, and long for the day when all lives really do matter equally.

Dinah and John W

John W lived five doors away from me in Finsbury Park. He had been diagnosed with Asperger's late in life and, looking back, he felt that his condition had made him a better engineer and a worse husband and father. Shortly after I met him he acquired a rescue dog from Battersea Dogs Home, and he and his little Max became a familiar sight in the neighbourhood, often stopping to chat and always friendly.

We would meet for lunch – Max tucked in quietly beside him – and discuss all manner of things. He was kind, clever and sociable, with firm and sometimes controversial views on politics, history, architecture, culture.

When I introduced him to Dinah, they got on well. John started to talk about his days in the army.

'I have no empathy,' he declared. He proceeded to recount in great detail an incident that he found fascinating but which was distressing to listen to. At that point Dinah closed her eyes, shrinking visibly as if she was in actual physical discomfort, and begged him to stop. This was to me reminiscent of the blog cited above – a case of 'feeling too much'. You might say that her capacity for empathy caused her temporarily to implode.

Here then were two people of almost identical demographic credentials, sharing a neurotype, yet reacting to the same story in polar-opposite ways. I reminded myself at that point to ignore generalisations about autism and empathy.

I am also reminded that the capacity for empathy can change from day to day, among all of us. I know this in myself and I have also witnessed it in Danny. When hearing of the melt-downs in which he is violent, you might judge him to be impervious to the feelings of others, seeing them only as objects (as per the stereotype that persists about autistic people). And yet, when not overwhelmed with his own distress, he has some-times shown an extraordinary level of sensitivity to the feelings that others are experiencing. This happens without words, without knowledge of any backstory, as if other people's distress comes off them like a scent or an aura that needs no verbal explanation. He has on several occasions been particularly affec-tionate to me, as to Corey and to Sarah, at times of our inner turmoil, touching us, looking into our eyes, being especially tender and gentle. He can come across as amusingly abrupt sometimes in demanding a toy instead of saying hello, or barg-ing past someone as if they don't exist – and yet he shows us time and time again that he cares, that he is concerned, and that he is sensitive to our distress.

So what are we left with, if we are to continue to unite so many people under one diagnostic label? If they differ so strongly amongst themselves, in characteristics as well as opin-ions, will there ever be the possibility of a common cause? While they may unite against some of the barriers that confront them all – lack of understanding, say, or failure to make reason-able adjustments for their needs – is it sensible, let alone viable, to try to find some unifying attributes or goals beyond these general aspirations? Why wouldn't autistic people be as varied as neurotypicals?

All I really hope is that even if disagreements are inevitable, they can co-exist and be debated without venom, name-calling and hostility.

39

THE FUTURE OF AUTISM

Autism is evolving, or, to put it another way – as I said in my doctoral thesis – trying to pin it down is like trying to pin down a cloud. It seems to exist, indeed it *does* exist, for a while, but it is permanently on the move and changing shape, and one day it may turn into something else or disappear altogether.

Danny's lifetime has coincided with a rapid development in knowledge of autism, but at the same time we still lack a shared understanding of its biological nature or how it should be regarded.

In Danny's thirty years, genomic exploration of autism has mushroomed. We now know that there is no single gene that causes autism, nor even a handful of genes. In fact, over one hundred genes are now implicated in this 'polygenic' condition, and many of these genes are 'de novo mutations' (changes that take place spontaneously, not derived from the parents' own genetic makeup). Instead, researchers postulate an intricate interplay of genetic and environmental factors, without being any clearer than they were when Danny was first diagnosed about what these factors are. Nor have researchers found a reliable 'biomarker' (for example a blood test, or an observable feature of the brain) to establish autism as a biological entity.

Nonetheless, a colossal and expensive scientific search goes on, alongside a parallel debate about the purpose and justification for it. In the case of genomic research, critics suggest that it may either prove fruitless or be misused, or both. For example, might the presence of a range of candidate genes be used as an inappropriately blunt instrument in antenatal decision-making? (Even people with the same single-gene condition can have wildly different outcomes, so a cluster of implicated genes would be an even more unpredictable basis for choosing or discarding a potential life.) Likewise, plans to maintain a large database of genetic information about autistic people are not universally welcomed. A storm of protest in the UK led to the (temporary) halting of the Spectrum 10K project at Cambridge University.[1]

Meanwhile, in the absence of organic tests for autism, clinical diagnosis still relies on how a person presents, in terms of the behavioural criteria set out in the DSM or ICD. And these criteria are under continual review, and generate further debate.

In 2013, the American Psychiatric Association produced a new definition of autism. No longer were Asperger syndrome and high-functioning autism two separate entities. Both were now merged, under the single category of autism spectrum disorder (ASD). Gone was the triad of impairments. Instead, autism would now consist of just two core domains: social communication deficits and repetitive behaviours.[2]

These changed criteria are easier to remember than their predecessors, which is nice for laypeople. We only have two core domains to recite. But on the other hand, the new DSM introduced a whole set of supplementary criteria – additional co-occurring conditions and 'specifiers' that some, but not all, autistic people may also experience. These embrace mental health problems (e.g. anxiety and depression), medical problems (e.g. gastrointestinal disorder and epilepsy) and neurological differences (e.g. ADHD and Tourette's), and they allow a more precise analysis of the individual autistic person's particular presentation and needs. (Another distinction used in clinical diagnostics is 'prototypical' autism versus 'syndromic' autism.[3]) These subcategories may offer a useful signpost as to different types of help required.

However, they also pose even greater challenges than before about what a typical autistic person might be like, if indeed there is such a person.

When Danny was diagnosed, in 1996, a 'typical' autistic person was usually portrayed as a child – non-verbal, lost and isolated, learning disabled and distressed. The sorrowing toddler, the jigsaw with a piece missing, the foggy outline of a person unknown and unknowable. Nowadays, a 'typical' autistic person may more likely be the articulate teenager or adult, experiencing the world and thinking about things in a way that differs from how NTs perceive their environment, but nonetheless whole, intact, entitled. So I nowadays describe Danny as autistic *plus*. Autistic *plus* learning disabled, autistic *plus* someone who doesn't use words, autistic *plus* someone experiencing additional health complications and behaviours that can sometimes be dangerous (to self or others).

I don't mind having to describe Danny, and people like him, as autistic plus, but some others do. Echoing the 'treatment vs acceptance' debate discussed in Chapter 23, these others feel that autism has been appropriated by a more intellectually able and vocal group who (it is alleged) wrongly claim sole representation of all autistics, and who thereby leave those with additional challenges sidelined and neglected. A recent statement authored by several of the Big Names proposes that the more disabled and complex group might benefit from the label 'profound autism'.[4] The proposal – along with so much within the autism world – has been welcomed by some and criticised by others.[5]

It is tempting to sympathise with those who want a distinct category for autistic people whose needs present the greatest challenge, to them and to others. Certainly, the intellectually disabled and minimally verbal group is under-researched.[6] This may not just be because they are less interesting to scientists, but rather because it is hard to enlist the cooperation necessary for testing. For example, MRI scans that are used to identify brain differences in autistic people require a level of comprehension and cooperation that would be intolerable and impossible for an autistic person like Danny. Nor will he be able to respond to questionnaires or general enquiries about his feelings and thoughts. Through observation, and knowledge of his distinct communication style and eloquent behaviour patterns, we know his opinion on different T-shirts and jigsaw puzzles, but these are not the topics that preoccupy scientists.

It seems that the research community is finally taking note. The pendulum may be swinging back to the point where experiences of learning-disabled autistics may be regarded as important questions in their own right.[7] And in the USA, the National Institutes of Health have recently put out a call specifically for research into the 'minimally verbal' group.[8]

Where do I stand in all of this?

I broadly welcome the range of specifiers introduced in 2013. I hope they might assist people to address distinct, additional challenges, rather than seeing all of autism as a target for treatment. I also welcome moves to attend to the learning disabled and minimally verbal. But a term like 'profound autism' is not the answer, because it is still an umbrella that ignores the necessary subtleties of individual difference. If you were to witness Danny's eye contact and his ability to cope with change, you might say that his autism is far less profound than that of a brilliant and articulate autistic mathematician who can only get through life by adhering every day to the same, rigid rituals.

Where I believe the drive to subcategorise autism may have most validity for broader application is in the field of education and social support, rather than in the biomedical sphere. We still need robust scientific research, but its focus should shift to things that can affect a person's progress significantly – learning style, teaching methods, the impact of environment and wider policy on individual progress – all with a view to maximising the life chances of autistic and 'autistic plus' people. This kind of enquiry seems to be less exciting to research funders unfortunately, and perhaps also to the wider scientific community, despite several reports that have called for this change of focus for decades.[9]

I believe that in education, health and social care, in both research and practice, a greater focus on individual difference could help depolarise some of the ideological and professional struggles that have plagued the field during Danny's life. In social care, it is obvious that what Danny needs to support him round the clock is profoundly different from the support that many able autistics require – reasonable adjustments in the workplace, for example. And in education, at a very obvious level, it may mean we could live with the assertion that any teaching approach and any educational setting – mainstream/ special school/home education – can be 'right' for some and 'wrong' for others. If so, we can welcome a variety of approaches as long as they are underpinned with a commitment to doing the best for each person, and an understanding that each individual's 'good outcome' may be unique to them.

This seems obvious to me, but unfortunately the debates still rage, and can be toxic and violent. Is there any hope of calming down these 'culture wars',[10] in which polar positions are taken with little room for discussion?

Yes, I have some hope about this, as a result of direct experience and recent discoveries.

In 2019, I was approached by Robert Chapman to co-write a chapter for a textbook on autism. Robert is a fellow postdoctoral ethics scholar, and the chapter for which he had been commissioned was about neurodiversity and the 'anti-therapy'

movement – which we felt had particular resonance around the
ABA controversy. We had originally met because we were the
only two people we knew of who were writing doctoral theses
about autism and ethics. While I brought twenty-plus years of
experience of how an autistic person like Danny, with severe
learning difficulties, gets through each day, Robert brought his
firsthand lifelong experience as an autistic person with a powerful intellect and extensive knowledge of philosophy.

We acknowledged in our chapter that as co-authors writing
about the ethics of ABA with regard to autism, one of us
favoured abolition, while the other favoured reform.[11] We
managed to collaborate with mutual respect and appreciation.
We discussed our divergent perspectives and challenged one
another, finding common ground in some places though not in
all, and, most importantly, highlighted areas that require deeper
conversation and further research. We agreed to disagree, and
did not try to shout the other person down, or prevent them
from airing their views.

And today, as I finalise the manuscript for the book, my inbox
brings me an article entitled 'Building bridges: Collaboration
across the autism community'.[12] I read of people who might
otherwise disagree managing to air their differences without
vitriol, while also uniting about the need for more, and better,
services and supports.

We need more of these collaborations. Given the existence of
the 'double empathy' problem, referred to in the previous chapter, I feel it may be particularly challenging for all of us in the
autism community to air disagreements politely and
respectfully.

So we need to be extra vigilant with regard to unconscious
bias, power imbalance or attempts to monopolise kudos and
influence. Patient and attentive listening, with as many adjustments to 'normal' debating forums as may be necessary in order
to build trust, could produce fruitful and truly reciprocal

exchange. And with this in mind, let me introduce you to one of the most interesting academic papers on autism I have read, once again with Dinah at the forefront.

Before she died, Dinah was involved in an exercise in which she, with one NT and two autistic academic colleagues, explored what they had in common and how they differed. The result – an important academic paper – describes a method for facilitating discussion and, in the process, learning more about autism and how we can all come to understand one another better. It also illuminates areas of commonality – including the need for human connection – and of difference (for example sensory processing). If lay readers want to read just one article, I suggest this is the one: 'The Human Spectrum: A Phenomenological Enquiry within Neurodiversity' (authored by Dinah Murray, Damian Milton, Jonathan Green and Jo Bervoets).[13] I ask readers unfamiliar with the term 'phenomenological' not to be put off (it basically means subjective experience of the world). Likewise, I ask scientists who usually prefer more traditional research methods (systematic observation and measurement) to rise above their scepticism.

So there are signs that people are willing to engage in conversations across the great divide. Oh, this is so long overdue. Why should any of us fight such battles with one another, at a time when our common cause is to campaign for better support, more generous funding, a professionalised social care workforce and robust systems of accountability? Should we not be joining forces against the greatest outrage of all – that autistic and learning-disabled people are being incarcerated in institutions far away from their communities, where they may be vulnerable to abuse, neglect and avoidable death? How many more exposés do there have to be before the system is radically overhauled?[14] In this wider context, intersectional debates can sometimes feel like a terrible and diversionary expenditure of outrage and intellectual energy.

But there is one area that is crying out for more attention. For obvious reasons, the process involved in Dinah's and colleagues' research was only accessible to autistic people with high intellect and communication skills. Such an exercise would not have been possible for autistic participants who are minimally verbal and intellectually disabled. And it was one of the authors – Jonathan Green – who has since stressed that not enough is yet known about intellectual disability, and that it should be a discrete focus for research.[15]

It is here that my key concern remains.

40

VALUING LEARNING DISABILITY

In my doctoral thesis I wrote about the danger of singling out the disabled when making public-expenditure arguments, and suggested that there is an ableist bias. For example, I wrote that we do not question the provision of street lighting even though it is an avoidable expense for blind people; the investment in public spending on sports facilities and treating sports injuries doesn't trigger a public outcry concerning the economic burden of physical activity. So I concluded that the choice of what are considered to be necessary and 'normal' areas of public expenditure, as opposed to avoidable and burdensome areas, is a political one that reflects underlying power structures and priorities about who are legitimate beneficiaries in our economy – and who are not.[1]

Echoing this, I worry that in research and in public policy, a line will be drawn between the section of the autistic population who are able to be economically or culturally productive – through employment, writing, art, etc. – and those who will be forever dependent on publicly funded support. Whereas many autistics can be gainfully employed (and more could be, with the right attitudes and adaptations), Danny and his minimally verbal, learning-disabled peers are entirely dependent on benefits and the NHS or local authorities to pay the wages of their support teams. (Either this, or their family members soldier on unassisted until the point of collapse.)

In what ways does the distinction between able and less able autistics matter, and in what areas is it a dangerous distraction? I believe there are two key points to make, one related to economics and the other to notions of the good life.

A crude belief that the learning disabled have nothing to contribute, while able autistics are welcome in our world (though only insofar as they are economically and culturally productive), underpins much of what has been written about the economic implications of autism and disability in general. There is a deep-rooted ideological component to all of this, which is based in prejudices rather than facts. The most obvious example is Nazi Germany, where propaganda was used to justify the extinction of disabled people *because they represented an economic drain*, even while catastrophically damaging and costly expenditure on rearmament was applauded. This is double-think at its most extreme. But something similar, though thankfully less murderous, still lurks below the surface of much contemporary 'liberal' thought. In the long run, I fear economic arguments may drive efforts to prevent some types of disability. They focus exclusively on the cost of supporting people who are not economically independent, and in so doing they ignore other factors.

First, they omit to consider that these may well be the lives that inflict least harm on others. Danny is never going to hack someone's email, launch an internet scam, cheer on warmongers or intimidate asylum seekers. He is not going to waste millions of pounds on vanity projects and ambitious schemes that turn out to be white elephants, nor indulge in corruption that ensures his friends benefit from lucrative backhanders. Weapons of mass destruction were not invented by people with learning disabilities.

Second, the fact that the money spent on Danny goes primarily towards employing people, who in turn stimulate the economy through their purchases and their own contributions to taxation, seems to be overlooked in notions of economic 'burden'. These judgements are made without reference to the wider circular flow of income in which we all both contribute and receive. They also reflect a mindset that sees spending on human welfare as somehow unproductive. While there may not be a 'magic money tree',[2] neither is there a fixed and finite amount of money that has to be rationed. If there were, we would all be getting poorer and poorer as the world population expanded, requiring each person to receive a small and smaller slice of the non-expanding cake. The history of economic growth manifestly disproves this myth.

Another reason to fear a crude division between the 'able' and 'less able' sections of the autistic population is that it leads to simplistic and inaccurate generalisations about whose lives are worthwhile and who suffers more. To explain this, I take you back to the research study (touched on in Chapter 35) that points to a correlation between the suicidality of adults with autism and the extent to which they have attempted, over a lifetime, to camouflage their autistic behaviours – in effect to 'pretend' to be neurotypical.[3]

This is so important.

It suggests that attempts to divert people from being autistic, or to hide the extent of their differences, can have fatal consequences. It is a key argument for advocating acceptance of neurodiversity, and for questioning some of the ways in which people are pressured to conform in order to gain social acceptance. It also hints at an area in which the learning disabled may be far less troubled than more able autistics. Camouflaging is a non-starter for Danny. Pretending to be normal has never been a goal. Rather, it is *because* he is so evidently disabled that he can access support and additional help. For people like Danny, the focus of any intervention is to foster learning, to open new horizons, to teach skills that will promote their ability to choose and exercise as much autonomy as is compatible with their safety – none of which is equivalent to becoming more 'normal'. Unlike more able autistics, he is protected and looked after, not preoccupied with how he appears to others or burdened with social expectations that he can't meet.

There is a bigger debate to be had here about the values that drive our political economy, one that goes to the core of liberal welfare-state democracies. National insurance principles are based on the idea that life contains risk, and that misfortunes and disadvantages of many kinds are primarily the result of random forces of luck (where you're born and to whom) and only marginally the result of differences in individual qualities. In the knowledge that any one of us may at some point be amongst the less fortunate, and that this is often beyond our control, we contribute to a universal safety net. The good sense in this relates to self-interest as well as fairness. I can see no persuasive argument to exclude the learning disabled from this safety net.

So I have tried to explain why neither the economic burden argument nor the quality of life argument are strong enough to justify value judgements about different 'types' of autism. I understand those who are alarmed by what they perceive to be the most 'extreme' manifestations of autistic and learning disabled distress, which – it can sometimes seem – no amount of environmental adaptation or understanding can allay. The damage that people have done to themselves and/or others, and the extreme vulnerability of these people, is certainly nothing to be celebrated. I am not calling for complacency. But my point is that it is not possible to correlate this in any straightforward way with a crude able/disabled divide. Moreover, it may well be that the most distressing extremes can be prevented in the future through improvements in the skills and understanding of people around them.

I also think we need to separate the things that are genuinely losses for the individuals themselves from those that just seem to onlookers to be a deprivation. I think limited ability to express oneself in a way that others will understand is one such real loss, because it can lead to great distress and – as with Danny – be dangerous, for example preventing the identification of serious medical problems. This to me is a legitimate focus for intervention, but there are other things that are far less problematic.

One such area is surely the issue of dependency. I consider that independence is an overblown ideal. We are all interdependent. The wealthiest, most seemingly autonomous person is still incredibly needy – of farmers, sewage workers, transport workers, builders and so on – not just within their own geographical vicinity but globally. We may value choice and autonomy, but let us not confuse this with independence.

Even though some profoundly disabled autistic people suffer or appear to have a diminished quality of life, this has to be set against all the ways in which others with a similar level of impairment can enjoy their lives and find contentment. Eva Kittay's wonderful phrase 'capacity for joy'[4] may well be something that many learning-disabled citizens have in greater abundance than do the rest of us. I believe that the consequences of seeking to belittle or remove the learning disabled as a category of people are far graver than the costs involved in caring for, nurturing and trying to maximise their life chances. Someone might want to do an economic model to try to prove or disprove this, but I can promise you they won't be able to factor in all the relevant variables – including the value of love and joy.

41

How Things Are Now

It is an entirely open question for me as to whether the *thing* that is autism may one day be pinned down – or, alternatively, reconceptualised entirely – through a mixture of empirical and analytical endeavour. And it remains to be seen how far the different wings of the autism movement can find some kind of peace.

However, I believe that all of us whose lives are touched by these questions are actually engaged in a bigger struggle. This is the struggle to elevate the kind, patient and caring over the grudging, judgemental and mean. The struggle to put more effort into understanding others, and less into labelling, criticising and condemning. The struggle to bridge differences in the spirit of mutual tolerance and curiosity, even to a place of mutual celebration.

Because of this, I suspect that my contribution to all these other debates may now be over. There are struggles that lie ahead for Danny and me, but the struggles of thought and belief that have accompanied our personal journey, a bit like the hard shoulder on the motorway, may now have come to an end. I don't know if I have anything more to say about these important issues.

To conclude, then, I will bring you back to Danny and to the people we have met along the road.

★

For the past ten years, Danny has been living a short walk away, at the midpoint between Nick and me. He is supported round the clock in his own one-bedroom flat and has access to a lovely communal garden with an all-important swing. He shares the building with other adults with learning disabilities, all of whom have their own tenancies, courtesy of Islington Council, and their own bespoke level of support, courtesy of a team employed by Centre 404 – a local learning disability and autism charity. He is in the heart of the community where he has lived all his life, close to shops, buses, parks and a local pub whose staff and regular patrons know him well. When so many learning-disabled and autistic adults are sent hundreds of miles away from their families and their communities, sometimes to a place of neglect or abuse, I know we have notched up yet another stroke of good fortune.

And he is still surrounded by his band of angels. Sarah, now a mother as well as a nurse, acts as Danny's social secretary in charge of his Facebook page. She was also his specialist caterer, managing to prepare batches of delicious biscuits from the minuscule range of ingredients that Danny's fragile gut was able to tolerate until we had to introduce a liquid-only diet.

John lives two minutes away, and is playing a crucial role in the features of Danny's care that require meticulous nursing oversight. In addition, you will regularly find John supporting Danny at the local pub, to spend time with Nick and with Danny's younger brothers Lowell and Jesse. You might also find Danny hanging out at another bar a few miles east, in the marina where Corey's boat is moored and where Danny often stays. There, guided and protected by Corey, he has had the

freedom to build an additional and independent social life and
fan base.

Other friendships have sustained and grown in our corner of
North London.

Donna loves her flat in Holloway, where her daughters visit
frequently, and Paul watches over them all, driving between his
home in Suffolk and his job in Spitalfields. Within a two-mile
radius you will also find Michele, Jack and Ben – all still Arsenal
season-ticket holders.

Further afield, now, you will come across Lee and his partner
Aude. In Scotland, where Dinah moved in 2020, her autistic
offspring Fergus has their own body of work on autism.[1] Larry
remains in Coventry, planting trees and chairing his local Labour
Party. The Storey family are still in Essex, where Michael has
continued to work night shifts to keep a roof over the head of
his sons. Ben completed various IT courses and learned to drive
and to speak and read Japanese, while still battling mightily to
get his entitlement to disability benefit reinstated. He is hoping
to complete a network engineering degree.

Sam is engaged to be married, and – until the Covid-19
pandemic struck – worked at Stansted Airport. He is now a
plumber and will soon have completed his retraining to acquire
all the necessary certificates.

Also dispersed from North London are the founding
TreeHouse pupils and trustees. All are well. Inevitably, Katharine
and Karen went on to set up a successor charity – CareTrade
– and Karen remains its indefatigable chief executive officer.

Su continues to be a mover and shaker in the world of bespoke
tailoring, while Elliot – as sunny and enthusiastic as ever – has a
steady part-time job at the local Premier Inn. One of the most
positive people I have ever met, Elliot is emphatically not within
the category of people with post-traumatic stress disorder
following ABA. I do not negate the experiences of those for
whom ABA was traumatic, but I would ask that they, in turn, do

not negate how well things have turned out for Elliot and many others – people who may remember their education and their tutors with warmth and appreciation, but keep their heads below the parapet and have no desire to come under fire.

Danny continues to weather his storms with steady equanimity. Yes he still experiences pain too often, and has endured various crises involving intermittent hospital care, but he soldiers on with maturity and enjoys the good times all the more. He still loves swings, the hammock in my garden, the music and puzzles and photos on his iPad, his picture books and soft toys. He will still requisition sets of keys, and seize people's mobile phones in a quest to find Fireman Sam on YouTube. And he goes on reminding us that a diagnosis of autism and learning disability may tell you rather little about a person. He still belies the textbooks and raises doubts about the relevance of traditional measures for assessing quality of life.

Take, for example, his relationship with Toby. They have continued to meet regularly and respond to one another with mutual tenderness and sensitivity, touching each other, looking into one another's eyes, smiling. This friendship would not show up in a long-term research study, which counts things like paid employment or having a life partner as signs of a good outcome, and deems alternatives to these norms to be – by definition – suboptimal. But aside from the anxiety about their health that those around them carry, Danny and Toby truly flourish. They have nice homes and meaningful relationships, even if they need two-to-one support for most aspects of their life and are unable to use words to communicate.

When I look at what others go through, I know that Danny and I have been gifted a panoply of luck. The cushion of support, financial security, meeting particular people at particular times, not to mention the wisdom of professionals in a sensible local authority – all this has led Danny to a sustainable level of well-being, for as long as his intestines hold out.

In addition to the specifics of our own good luck, I also believe there is room for hope more generally. For example, I discovered the following journal extract:

Everywhere there is kindness.

What Danny has brought with him is access to an ocean of goodwill.

The shopkeepers who wanted to give him an extra bag of crisps free of charge, the fairground workers who would allow him to stay on the same ride time after time, the ladies in the café who told me not to apologise for him, not ever, when he screamed and banged and disturbed their lunch break. The nurses, the doctors, the teachers. The support workers who manage his periodic outbursts and attacks, who empty his stoma bag, who wash his soiled laundry if it bursts, who delight in his pleasures and are thrilled when he learns to run his own bath and wipe the table, who come back day after day to be with him and rub his feet as he goes through hours of pain, and whose hearts sing when he greets them with a look and a smile, a touch, a hug.

I have learned that most people are just waiting for a chance to be nice. For all the perpetrators of hate crimes, bullying, neglect and indifference, there are many, many more individuals whose everyday kindnesses and sense of decency win through. We don't read about this much, it's rarely on the news, and it doesn't make for dramatic TV series or interesting reality TV shows. But there it is.

And around every corner, in every child, there is the potential to be a human who isn't tarnished and whose values aren't distorted through commercial pressures and a toxic environment of competition and division.

It shines out in the way people catch Danny's innocence and enjoy his freedom from all that trash. They want to help

him to stay safe, to thrive in his way and *on his terms*. Kindness
is everywhere, in and around us, just waiting to shine.

This I know.

I know too that those words were written at a point in time
that may not come again. That the army of care workers and
health workers, whose sole purpose is to bring help and hope
to those they serve, are under enormous pressure; they are
undervalued, underpaid and often invisible in our strange
society with its fixation on ownership and acquisition and its
off-beam notions of 'success'. And there are not enough of
them.

I know that Danny's well-being has been hard won, and is
thanks chiefly to all those who have journeyed with him. For all
that he has cost the NHS a lot of money, and Nick a whole load
too, Danny has touched, inspired and indeed employed a large
team of people who believe in what they do, and who believe
in him. He has brought forth kindness, and in so doing he has
drawn attention to how plentiful this human quality can be, not
simply among those employed in caring jobs, but among all
types of people who would otherwise have little opportunity to
exercise this most essential of human qualities.

If only we could melt the iceberg of conflict that has
obstructed the safe passage of autistic people, their ideas and
learning over too many years. If only responses to learning disability – from education, social and health care, and from the
media – were higher up the political agenda. If only we could
bust the myth that public expenditure on human welfare is
some kind of subversive add-on to the 'real' business of uncon-
trolled private markets.

I have learned also that a whole array of widely accepted
accolades or markers of success cannot touch the achievements
of a man like Danny, who has been brave and stoical and patient
and trusting, full of humour and able to enjoy all the good

things that come his way, and somehow gets through the pain
without bitterness or self-pity.

★

Finally, I wish to share with you the question that Danny – and
all the people he has led me to meet – has posed ever since I
first realised he was never going to be 'normal'. The question is
as follows.

What kind of species do we humans want to become?

I started to write this section in early 2020, while Australia
burned and Greta Thunberg berated the powerful for having
done so little about climate change. Since then we have experienced more fires – Western USA, Moria refugee camp, Siberia,
Turkey, Greece, the Amazon rainforest – not to mention floods,
volcanic eruptions, a pandemic and terrible wars. No doubt
more will rage before this book sees the light of day.

The planet will survive in whatever form, but many species
will not. Sadly, it seems that we are not designed to cope very
well with our own ability to destroy so much that is precious,
despite my previous eulogy to the kindness that Danny has
drawn out in so many ordinary people. If you follow the arguments put forward by some philosophers,[2] humans are not
equipped with sufficient resources of altruism. We are too
self-interested and too short-termist in our thinking. We don't
give enough consideration to the needs of future generations
– we are numb to their potential suffering. If we are to survive,
they say, we need to extend our capacity for sympathy and
concern beyond our immediate circle and beyond our own
limited lifespan. The analysis leads these philosophers to advocate 'moral enhancement' – by pharmacological means if necessary – if our entire species is to be saved from self-destruction.

In response, I wonder if it is truly our moral failings or,
instead, the failings of political and economic systems, that have

led to the current state of peril. Or perhaps it is the result of a self-reinforcing cycle in which our natures drive the kinds of social institutions and structures that emerge, and these in turn influence the kind of people we become.

I believe there is an interplay. I believe too that the question of how we should evolve is not a merely hypothetical one. The technological army marches on, along with the quest of genomic science to eliminate certain types of intolerable diseases. Some conditions may be so horrid that we are well rid of them. But will the heady drive to predict, and prevent, other types of human variation take us further, into a eugenic dystopia?

'After a shift,' said Aaron, a recent member of Danny's entourage, 'I feel charged up with positive energy, like he's deleted some of the pessimism from the world, or from me.'

I embrace the idea of a future world where more people like Danny inspire more people like Aaron to feel this way. These are the things that make us human.

Whether we are anticipating a Brave New World, a Gattaca future, a Blade Runner universe or seeing only the world we currently inhabit – where the vast majority of Down syndrome foetuses are aborted and the disabled are often viewed with pity at best, and fear and resentment frequently – we need to take a very long, hard look at ourselves. What kinds of humanity do we promote, what kinds of humanity do we discard, and why? If society chooses to withhold support – support that it is perfectly capable of providing – to certain groups of vulnerable people, what does this say about the kind of people running it? What has become of us? And what or who will we become?

So here I bow out, done with preaching. Instead, it is Danny who claims the last words, via an excerpt from my journal written in the autumn of 2016.

Last night, the text I got from John at 9.15 p.m. after a day of pain, said this:

*'Dan's just walked into the lounge naked, grinning from
ear to ear, holding a flashing disco ball. All is well again. X'*

All those years ago, I would never have known that this
image, this precise image, is what I would want more than
anything for my twenty-three-year-old son. That it would
bring more tender grace than any number of glamorous
professions or heroic deeds – the aspirations that perhaps
other mothers may have for their young men. And sure, if
my glass were half empty, I could observe that he is ignoring
the learning he's acquired about the necessity of wearing
clothes when in the lounge. Not due to a slavish adherence
to social norms, but so that he will be less vulnerable in the
future if he knows that nakedness is only OK in private.

But to be sidetracked at this point would miss the beauty
and truth of the moment. Right now, in the context of
John's text, the nakedness is an expression of exuberance
and exultant liberation from the chains of pain, the medi-
cated fog, of recent days. And it is also a statement of
self-affirmation:

*This is me, look at me, I'm happy with my body with its scars
and stoma bag and I'm thrilled by my fabulous disco ball with its
colours and lights. I want to share this joyful moment with you, my
dear friend.*

This is who I am.

Smile with me.

Rejoice with me.

NOTES

1 DANNY

1. Danny's appreciation of affection was something that led some people to assert, later on, that he couldn't be autistic. In fact, what it meant was that those who held this view were merely echoing anecdotes that had mutated into hard, damaging and misleading generalisations and falsehoods about autism.
2. Lack of joint attention was cited as a key difference between autistic and typically developing toddlers. See, for example, Simon Baron-Cohen, *Autism and Asperger syndrome: The Facts*. Oxford: OUP (2008).

2 AN INTRODUCTION TO AUTISM

1. World Health Organization, International Statistical Classification of Diseases and Related Health Problems. Geneva: WHO (1992); American Psychiatric Association, Diagnostic and Statistical Manual of Mental Disorders. (4th edn) Washington, DC: APA (2000).
2. The triad of impairments related to impairments in social interaction, communication and interaction. See Lorna Wing, *The Autistic Spectrum: A Guide for Parents and Professionals*. London: Constable & Robinson (1996).

3.   An important account of how stimming has been misun-
     derstood in the past, but then reclaimed by autistic people,
     is: Steven K. Kapp, Robyn Steward, Laura Crane, Daisy
     Elliott et al., '"People should be allowed to do what they
     like": Autistic adults' views and experiences of stimming'.
     Autism, 2019, 23 (7), pp. 1,782–92.

4.   The term 'cognitive disability' is also adopted as an alterna-
     tive to 'learning disability' and 'intellectual disability'. 'Mental
     retardation', 'feeble-minded', 'imbecile' and so on have all
     been superseded with terms that are deemed to be more
     respectful. For further exploration of these issues, see Simon
     Jarrett, *Those They Called Idiots: The Idea of the Disabled Mind
     from 1700 to the Present Day*. London: Reaktion Books (2020).

5.   This theory examined difficulties in 'mind-reading' – in the
     sense of understanding that others' mental states have a
     separate existence from one's own, that other people may
     have different thoughts, beliefs, desires and intentions. For a
     contemporary critique of the proposition, see Sue Fletcher-
     Watson and Francesca Happé, *Autism: A New Introduction to
     Psychological Theory and Current Debate*. Abingdon: Routledge
     (2019), Chapter 6.

6.   The weak central coherence (WCC) thesis of autism
     ascribes autistic behaviours to a failure to see the whole,
     with a corresponding hyperfocus on details. Adherents of
     the WCC model feel it explains factors associated with
     autism that are not associated with mind-reading. See
     Fletcher-Watson and Happé, *Autism*, pp. 122–6.

7.   Executive function enables an individual to plan and organ-
     ise, by overriding automatic behaviours, inhibiting inappro-
     priate impulsive actions and resolving conflicting responses
     (Uta Frith, *Autism: Explaining the Enigma*. (2nd edn) Oxford:
     Blackwell (2003), pp. 177–8).

8.   See, for example, the discussion on monotropism (note 6,
     Chapter 23) and recent developments (Chapters 38 and 39).

9. See Sami Timimi, Neil Gardner and Brian McCabe, *The Myth of Autism: Medicalising Men's Social and Emotional Competence.* Basingstoke: Palgrave Macmillan (2011); David G. Amaral, Geraldine Dawson and Daniel H. Geschwind (eds), *Autism Spectrum Disorders.* New York: Oxford University Press (2011).

10. In particular, Clara Claiborne Park, *The Siege.* New York: Harcourt, Brace & World (1967); Catherine Maurice, *Let Me Hear Your Voice: A Family's Triumph Over Autism.* New York: Random House (1993).

11. Temple Grandin, *Thinking in Pictures: My Life with Autism.* (Expanded edition) New York: Vintage (2006).

12. Donna Williams, *Nobody Nowhere: The Remarkable Autobiography of an Autistic Girl.* London: Jessica Kingsley Publishers (1998).

13. *Rain Man*, Barry Levinson, dir. (United Artists, 1988).

14. An enlightening account of Bettelheim's theory and practices, and critiques thereof, is contained in Chapter 3 of Adam Feinstein, *A History of Autism: Conversations with the Pioneers.* Chichester: Wiley-Blackwell (2010).

15. Bernard Rimland was one of the founders of the Autism Society of America (https://autism.wikia.org/wiki/Autism_Society_of_America), and author of *Infantile Autism: The Syndrome and Its Implications for a Neural Theory of Behavior*, New York: Appleton-Century-Crofts (1964), which postulated an organic rather than emotional explanation of autism.

16. A good overview of the research in these areas is contained in Chapter 4 of Fletcher-Watson and Happé, *Autism.*

3   No Man's Land

1. Saturday 6 December 1997, *Daily Telegraph Weekend*, article by Nick entitled 'Life with Danny'.

2. Mitzi Waltz, 'The Production of the "Normal" Child: Neurodiversity and the Commodification of Parenting' in Hanna Rosqvuist, Nick Chown, Anna Stenning (eds)

Neurodiversity Studies: A New Critical Paradigm. Abingdon: Routledge (2020).

3. See Fletcher-Watson and Happé, *Autism*, pp. 21–7.

4   KIDZMANIA

1. The social model of disability emphasises the environmental obstacles and prejudices that pervade society and asserts that disability is caused by these conditions, distinct from the impairment a disabled individual has. This is in contrast to the medical model, which presents disability purely as an individual's malfunction. The social model underpins *Fundamental Principles of Disability*, the foundational statement of the disability movement, adopted by the Union of the Physically Impaired Against Segregation (UPIAS) on 3 December 1974, amended 9 July 1976.

2. Equality Act 2010. London: The Stationery Office, available from: http://legislation.gov.uk/ukpga/2010/15/contents.

5   ON THE MARGINS

1. Charlotte Moore, *George and Sam*. London: Penguin Books (2012).

2. Pauline Heslop, Peter Blair, Peter Fleming, Matt Hoghton et al., *Confidential Inquiry into premature deaths of people with learning disabilities (CIPOLD)*. Norah Fry Research Centre: Bristol (2013); Sara Ryan, *Justice for Laughing Boy: Connor Sparrowhawk – A Death by Indifference*. London: Jessica Kingsley Publishers (2018).

3. Hate crimes against disabled people are exposed powerfully in Katharine Quarmby, *Scapegoat: Why We Are Failing Disabled People*. London: Portobello Books (2011).

4. Saba Salman (ed.), *Made Possible: Stories of success by people with learning disabilities – in their own words*. London: Unbound (2020).

7 EARLY INTERVENTION

1. See, for example, Lauren Nicolle, 'Thousands of Children with SEND unable to access formal education'. *Learning Disability Today*, 14 February 2024, available from: https://www.learningdisabilitytoday.co.uk/news/thousands-of-children-with-send-unable-to-access-formal-education/ [accessed 8 March 2024].

2. Instead read Catherine Maurice, *Let Me Hear Your Voice: A Family's Triumph Over Autism*. New York: Random House (1993) and Steve Silberman, *NeuroTribes: The Legacy of Autism and How to Think Smarter About People Who Think Differently*. London: Allen & Unwin (2015).

3. Research Autism was an independent charity prior to its merger with the UK's National Autistic Society. See https://www.informationautism.org/autism-interventions.

8 ABA: GOOD NEWS?

1. O. Ivar Lovaas, 'Behavioral treatment and normal educational and intellectual functioning in young autistic children'. *Journal of Consulting and Clinical Psychology*, 1987, 55, 3–9.

2. John J. McEachin, Tristram Smith and O. Ivar Lovaas, 'Long-Term Outcome for Children with Autism Who Received Early Intensive Behavioral Treatment'. *American Journal on Mental Retardation*, 1993, 97 (4), 359–72.

9 ABA: THE CONTROVERSY

1. Practices at the Judge Rotenberg Center (JRC) have been the subject of legal challenge and counter-challenge. The Autism Self Advocacy Network (ASAN) has campaigned strenuously for the practices to be banned. See, for example, 'ASAN Commends FDA's Move to Appeal Judge Rotenberg Center Ruling', available from: https://autisticadvocacy.org/2021/09/asan-commends-fdas-move-to-appeal-judge-

rotenberg-center-ruling/. Less widely known is the fact that several behaviour analysts and ABA groups are deeply critical of the JRC, and have themselves boycotted events at which it has been invited to present. See '900 ABA Professionals Have Weighed in on the Use of Electroshock at Judge Rotenberg Center', available from: https://neuroclastic. com/900-aba-professionals-have-weighed-in-on-the-use-of-electroshock-at-judge-rotenberg-cennter/.

2. A text I found helpful as a layperson trying to understand different models of ABA with regard to autism was Laura Schreibman, *The Science and Fiction of Autism*. London: Harvard University Press (2005). The field has developed and expanded considerably since then, as an internet search of different models of ABA will reveal.

3. TEACCH originally stood for 'Treatment and Education of Autistic and related Communications Handicapped Children'. It is still used in the UK in some schools.

10 TREEHOUSE

1. M.J. Maenner, Z. Warren, A.R. Williams, E. Amoakohene et al., 'Prevalence and Characteristics of Autism Spectrum Disorder Among Children Aged 8 Years – Autism and Developmental Disabilities Monitoring Network, 11 Sites, United States, 2020'. *MMWR Surveillance Summaries*, 2023, 72 (2), 1–14, available from: http://dx.doi.org/10.15585/mmwr.ss7202a1.

12 MARCHING

1. Autism Act 2009. London: The Stationery Office, available from: https://www.legislation.gov.uk/ukpga/2009/15/contents.

13 DONNA, DANIEL AND PAUL

1. A punchy commentary on the system is offered by *Special Needs Jungle* columnist Matt Keer, whose analysis of the

statistics around Special Educational Needs and Disability (SEND) tribunals highlights the inadequacy of many local authorities' processes and decision-making in the field of SEN. '95% of decisions in favour of parents, but nobody wins at the SEND Tribunal'. *Special Needs Jungle*, 11 December 2020. [Online], available from: https://www.specialneedsjungle.com/95-decisions-favour-parents-nobody-wins-send-tribunal/ [accessed 26 August 2021].

14 THE MMR CONTROVERSY

1. Andrew Wakefield, Simon Murch, Andrew Anthony, John Walker-Smith et al., 'RETRACTED: Ileal-lymphoid-nodular hyperplasia, non-specific colitis, and pervasive developmental disorder in children'. *The Lancet*, 28 February 1998, 351 (9103), 637–41, available from: https://www.thelancet.com/journals/lancet/article/PIIS0140-6736(97)11096-0/fulltext.

2. For a detailed account of the events, the science and the controversy, see Paul A. Offit, *Autism's False Prophets: Bad Science, Risky Medicine, and the Search for a Cure*. New York: Columbia University Press (2008).

15 MMR AND SIMON MURCH

1. Fabricated or Induced Illness is regarded in the UK as a form of child abuse and is a child safeguarding issue. See https://www.nhs.uk/mental-health/conditions/fabricated-or-induced-illness/overview/.

2. Allergy Induced Autism, or AIA, was a UK-based, parent-led group that promoted biomedical interpretations of autism, and was strongly aligned with the parents who litigated against the MMR drug companies. See Michael Fitzpatrick, *Defeating Autism: A Damaging Delusion*. Abingdon: Routledge (2009).

3. The debate was covered widely in the media. See, for example, Sarah Boseley, 'Doctors turn on each other as MMR debate rages again: Architects of autism study embroiled in bitter dispute', *Guardian*, 1 November 2003, available from: https://www.theguardian.com/society/2003/nov/01/highereducation.medicineandhealth.

16 COREY

1. 'Divorce among parents of children with autism: dispelling urban legends'. *Autism*, 2013, 17 (6), 643–4, available from: https://doi.org/10.1177/1362361313509528.

18 DEPRESSION AND IDENTITY

1. Andrew Solomon, *The Noonday Demon: An Atlas of Depression*. New York: Simon and Schuster (2001).
2. Lewis Wolpert, *Malignant Sadness: The Anatomy of Depression*. London: Faber and Faber (2001).
3. First Epistle of St Paul the Apostle to the Corinthians, Chapter 13.
4. Jim Sinclair, 'Don't Mourn for Us'. Autism Network International newsletter *Our Voice*, 1993, 1 (3), available from: http://www.autreat.com/dont_mourn.html.
5. Jon Adams in conversation with Steve Silberman at an event in London organised by the National Autistic Society in September 2015. (Sections of the event were posted on YouTube on 8 October 2015, though they don't include Jon's comment: https://www.youtube.com/watch?v=NFPNIBmqAHQ.)
6. Jackie Leach Scully, *Disability Bioethics: Moral Bodies, Moral Difference*. Plymouth: Rowman and Littlefield (2008).
7. Micheline Mason, *Incurably Human*. (2nd edn) Nottingham: Inclusive Solutions (2005).

19 DEBBIE

1. See his book *Disabled Children: A Legal Handbook* (2020) co-authored with Luke Clements and published by the Legal Action Group and the Council for Disabled Children (2020).

2. Mike Stanton, *Learning to Live with High Functioning Autism: A Parent's Guide for Professionals*. London: Jessica Kingsley Publishers (2000), p. 44.

3. See Matthew Chapman, 'Bestseller helps parents fight accusations of child abuse: Novel has shed light on Asperger's Syndrome but families still find themselves under investigation', *Guardian*, 26 September 2004, available from: https://www.theguardian.com/society/2004/sep/26/childrensservices.books, and his BBC coverage, 'Asperger's abuse inquiry pledged', 25 September 2004, available from http://news.bbc.co.uk/1/hi/health/3687612.stm.

4. Armorer Wason, *Constructive Campaigning for Autism Services: The PACE Parents' Handbook*. London: Jessica Kingsley Publishers (2005). The handbook includes the suggestion that a confrontational approach may in some situations be less persuasive than reasoned argument, if one is trying to persuade people in positions of power to change.

20 REFLECTIONS

1. Pre-implantation genetic testing (PGT) 'can be performed on cells from early embryos created by in vitro fertilisation (IVF) so that those with a particular genetic feature are not transferred into the uterus'. Royal College of Physicians, Royal College of Pathologists and British Society for Genetic Medicine, *Ethical issues in prenatal genetic diagnosis: Guidance for clinical practice*. Report of the Joint Committee on Genomics in Medicine. London: RCP, RCPath and BSGM (2022), p. 35, available from: https://www.rcplondon.ac.uk/projects/outputs/ethical-issues-prenatal-genetic-diagnosis.

2. See Sandy Starr, 'How to talk about genome editing'. *British Medical Bulletin*, June 2018, 126 (1), 5–12, available from: https://doi.org/10.1093/bmb/ldy015.
3. For example, Bob Wright. See Chapter 28.
4. For example, Allen Buchanan, Dan W. Brock, Norman Daniels and Daniel Wikler, *From Chance to Choice: Genetics & Justice*. New York, Cambridge: Cambridge University Press (2000).
5. See, for example, Julian Savulescu, 'Deaf Lesbians, "Designer Disability", and the Future of Medicine'. *British Medical Journal*, 2002, 325, 771–3.

22 Larry, and the Wider Autism Movement

1. For a brief overview of controversial treatments such as these, see Matt Carey, 'Scientists must curb tendency to try untested treatments', *Spectrum*, 12 May 2016, available from: https://www.spectrumnews.org/opinion/viewpoint/scientists-must-curb-tendency-to-try-untested-treatments/.

23 Tribalism

1. Jeremy Laurance, 'Autism: What are the ethics of treating disability? A row about the correct response to the condition – acceptance or treatment – is dividing campaigners and carers', *Independent*, 16 November 2007.
2. 8 November 2007 letter from Treating Autism. 10 November 2007 four letters: from Phil Culmer (autistic man), from Benet Middleton (National Autistic Society), from Celia Forrest (mother of autistic son) and from Geoffrey Maddrell (Research Autism). 14 November 2007 three letters: from Paul Wady (autistic man), from Doreen Carlson (mother of autistic son) and from Haywood Drake (autistic person). 17 November 2007 letter from Steph Sirr (mother of autistic son). 22 November 2007 letter from Angie Elliot (mother of autistic daughter).

3. Discussion between Richard Mills and original author of *Treating Autism* letter to the *Independent*. *Today*, BBC Radio 4. November 2007. [Radio broadcast].

4. Launched by the National Autistic Society (NAS) in October 2007.

5. Simon Baron-Cohen, *The Essential Difference: Men, Women and the Extreme Male Brain*. London: Penguin (2004).

6. Dinah Murray, Mike Lesser and Wendy Lawson, 'Attention, monotropism and the diagnostic criteria for autism'. *Autism*, 2005, 9 (2), 136–56.

7. Ibid. p. 142.

8. See Fletcher-Watson and Happé, *Autism*, a textbook that includes influential ideas generated by autistic authors (see especially Chapters 9 and 10) and a commentary at the end of each chapter by neurodivergent writers ('community contributors').

9. Saskia Baron, 'Autism unpacked: how my brother's autism has changed over 50 years and how the definition of autism as a whole has changed over his lifetime'. Presentation delivered at the NAS Professional Conference, held on 5–6 March 2013, Harrogate.

10. Amanda Baggs, *In My Language*. 2007, available from: https://www.youtube.com/watch?v=JnylM1hI2jc. Amanda Baggs also went by the name Mel Baggs (or sometimes Amelia Baggs) in later years.

11. This phrase underpins the importance of Augmentative and Alternative Communication (AAC), which an umbrella term for a range of tools that supplement or replace speech. These can be pictures, symbols and photos; signing and gestures; and speech-generating devices. See 'What is AAC?', *Communication Matters*, available from https://www.communicationmatters.org.uk/what-is-aac/. The use of AAC has been a significant help for learning-disabled people who struggle with spoken communication,

and in some cases enabled people who were previously written off as non-verbal, to demonstrate that they possess both cognitive and linguistic ability.

24 ABA Tribes and Michelle Dawson

1. Michelle Dawson, 'The Misbehaviour of Behaviourists: Ethical Challenges to the Autism-ABA Industry'. 2004. [Online], available from: https://www.sentex.ca/~nexus23/ naa_aba.html.
2. Details of the court case (Auton vs British Columbia) and Dawson's submission can be found on her website *No Autistics Allowed* here: https://www.sentex.ca/~nexus23/ naa_fac.html.
3. I am glad to note that sections of the ABA community do recognise the validity of these criticisms and are calling for change. See, for example, Megan S. Kirby, Trina D. Spencer and Shane T. Spiker, 'Humble Behaviorism Redux'. *Behavior and Social Issues*, 2022, available from: https://doi. org/10.1007/s42822-022-00092-4.
4. 'Challenges to autism intervention research: costs, benefits, problems and solutions', delivered on 28 February 2012 at the National Autistic Society Professional Conference – Working Together for Better Outcomes, held on 28–29 February 2012 in Manchester.
5. 'Campaigning for Autism Services: Reflections on the past, dreams for the future', delivered on 12 January 2012 at the Autism Spectrum Disorder: from clinical practice to educational provision conference held on 12–13 January 2012 at the Irish Centre for Autism and Neurodevelopmental Research, National University of Ireland, Galway.
6. See Tara Bannow, 'Parents and clinicians say private equity's profit fixation is short-changing kids with autism'. *STAT*, 15 August 2022. [Online], available from: https://www.

statnews.com/2022/08/15/private-equity-autism-aba-therapy/?utm_source=Spectrum+Newsletters&utm_campaign=d8ceb25035-EMAIL_CAMPAIGN_DAILY_20220816_TUESDAY&utm_medium=e-mail&utm_term=0_529db1161f-d8ceb25035-168640661.

7. I should also add that change is starting to happen in the USA. See, for example, Yev Veverka, 'Applied behavior analysis and autism: Flawed application of a proven science'. *Spectrum*, 1 September 2022, available from: https://www.spectrumnews.org/opinion/viewpoint/applied-behavior-analysis-and-autism-flawed-application-of-a-proven-science/?utm_source=Spectrum+Newsletters&utm_campaign=a0dc552884-EMAIL_CAMPAIGN_DAILY_20220901&utm_medium=email&utm_term=0_529db1161f-a0dc552884-168640661.

27 DINAH

1. See Jordan, Jones and Murray, *Educational Interventions for Children with Autism: A Literature Review of Recent and Current Research*. DfEE Research Report No. 77. London: DfEE (1998).

2. The acronym stood for Autistic People Against Neuroleptic Abuse. See Dinah Murray, 'Autistic People Against Neuroleptic Abuse', in Steven K. Kapp (ed.), *Autistic Community and the Neurodiversity Movement: Stories from the Frontline*. Singapore: Springer Nature (2020), 51–63.

3. Wendy Lawson, *Concepts of Normality: The Autistic and Typical Spectrum*. London: Jessica Kingsley Publishers (2008).

4. Dinah Murray, 'From Protest to Taskforce', in Kapp (ed.), *Autistic Community and the Neurodiversity Movement*, 277–85.

28 THE WRIGHTS AND RIGHTS

1. For Dinah's public, published account of these events, see ibid. 277–85.

2. Autism Speaks had 'cure' as part of its founding mission in 2005, but has since distanced itself from this goal. See, for example, Michelle Diament, 'Autism Speaks No Longer Seeking Cure', *Disability Scoop*, 14 October 2016, available from: https://www.disabilityscoop.com/2016/10/14/autism-speaks-no-longer-cure/22884/.
3. *Something About Us*, available from: https://www.youtube.com/watch?v=J-014P0hQ6w (Part 1) and https://www.youtube.com/watch?v=Dna1Z41_w3c (Part 2).
4. Jardine, 'Should we want to cure autism?'. *Telegraph*, 22 October 2008.
5. Inaugural TreeHouse annual lecture, 2008, featuring Bob Wright, Jon Snow, Anya Ustaszewski, Larry Arnold and me, available from: https://rightfullives.net/VideoPages/TreeHouse.html.
6. Pete Wharmby, *Untypical: How the world isn't built for autistic people and what we should all do about it*. London: Mudlark/HarperCollins (2023).
7. This was *Autism: Challenging Behaviour*, produced by Fran Robinson (BBC 4, 5 November 2013). Together with Bob Remington, I had been credited as a consultant, because I had encouraged Fran to address the ethical debate around ABA with regard to autism.
8. Concluding sentences of Sandy Starr's speech at the Autism, Ethics and Good Life conference, 2 April 2012. British Academy, London ksj – s.

29 GROUNDHOG YEARS
1. 'Picture Window', from the album *Lonely Avenue*, lyrics by Nick Hornby, music by Ben Folds (Nonesuch Records 79786, 2010).

30 LEE
1. Nick Hornby, *31 Songs*. London: Penguin (2002).

31 HELEN KEELER AND EUGENICS

1. Deborah R. Barnbaum, *The Ethics of Autism: Among Them, but Not of Them*. Bloomington: Indiana University Press (2008).

2. See note 5 in Chapter 2, p. 262.

3. See notes 6 and 7 in Chapter 2, p. 262.

4. Barnbaum, *The Ethics of Autism*, p. 64.

5. Joel Feinberg, 'The Child's Right to an Open Future', in William Aiken and Hugh LaFollette (eds), *Whose Child? Children's Rights, Parental Authority, and State Power*. Totowa, NJ: Rowman and Littlefield (1980), 124–53.

6. A full, technical discussion of Feinberg's argument is contained in Stephen Wilkinson, *Choosing Tomorrow's Children: The Ethics of Selective Reproduction*. Oxford: Oxford University Press (2010), 44–54.

7. Sarah Zhang, 'The Last Children of Down Syndrome'. *The Atlantic*, December 2020, available from: https://www.theatlantic.com/magazine/archive/2020/12/the-last-children-of-down-syndrome/616928/ [accessed 1 September 2021].

8. James Tapper, 'Fury at "do not resuscitate" notices given to Covid patients with learning disabilities', *Observer*, 13 February 2021, available from: https://www.theguardian.com/world/2021/feb/13/new-do-not-resuscitate-orders-imposed-on-covid-19-patients-with-learning-difficulties.

9. For example, Jeff McMahan, *The Ethics of Killing*. New York: Oxford University Press (2002); Peter Singer, *Animal Liberation*. London: Pimlico (1995).

34 HOME AND AWAY

1. Ari Ne'eman cited by Andrew Solomon, *Far From the Tree: A Dozen Kinds of Love*. London: Chatto & Windus (2013), p. 275.

2. Helen Keeler, 'Unnatural selection'. *BioNews*, 538, 14 December 2009, available from: https://www.bionews.org.uk/page_92061. See also my chapter 'Is There an Ethical

Case for the Prevention and/or Cure of Autism?' in Hanna Bertilsdotter Rosqvist, Nick Chown and Anna Stenning (eds), *Neurodiversity Studies: A New Critical Paradigm*. London: Routledge (2020).

3. IACC–NIH Workshop: Ethical, Legal and Social Implications (ELSI) of Autism Research – 26 September 2011. Slides available from: https://iacc.hhs.gov/meetings/autism-events/2011/oarc/september26/slides_elsi_092611.pdf.

4. For ASAN, see https://autisticadvocacy.org. ASAN, Symposium on Ethical, Legal and Social Implications of Autism Research. Held on 10 December 2011. Videos of proceedings available online from: https://www.youtube.com/watch?v=ziCsNWZmONA and https://www.youtube.com/watch?v=H1tPKN7alhw.

5. Ari Ne'eman, *The Right to Live in This World: The Untold Story of Disability in America*. New York: Simon & Schuster (2021).

6. Keise Izuma, Kenji Matsumoto, Colin F. Camerer and Ralph Adolphs, 'Insensitivity to social reputation in autism'. *Proceedings of the National Academy of Sciences*, 10 October 2011, 108 (42), 17302–7, available from: http://www.pnas.org/content/108/42/17302.full.

7. Elissar Andari, Jean-René Duhamel, Tiziana Zalla, Evelyn Herbrecht et al., 'Promoting social behaviour with oxytocin in high-functioning autism spectrum disorders'. *Proceedings of the National Academy of Sciences of the United States of America*, 2010, 107 (9), 4389–94.

8. Michelle Dawson, 'Oxytocin versus autism: A cure for altruism'. 17 February 2010. [Online], available from: http://autismcrisis.blogspot.co.uk/2010/02/oxytocin-versus-autism-cure-for.html.

35 SURGERY

1. I am aware of growing research into a possible connection between autism spectrum disorder, pain, hypermobility and

other connective tissue disorders. Here is just one example: Carolina Baeza-Velasco, David Cohen, Claude Hamonet, Elodie Vlamynck et al., 'Autism, Joint Hypermobility-Related Disorders and Pain'. *Frontiers in Psychiatry*, 7 December 2018, 9, Article 656, available from: https://doi.org/10.3389/fpsyt.2018.00656.

2. I am not aware of any ethical opposition to genetic treatment to tackle sickle-cell disease on the grounds of the impact on the ethnic group most affected. See, for example, Michael Eisenstein, 'Gene therapies close in on a cure for sickle-cell disease'. *Nature*, 25 August 2021, available from: https://www.nature.com/articles/d41586-021-02138-w [accessed 25 September 2021]. Likewise, in regard to thalassaemia, see A. Cao, C. Rosatelli, R. Galanello, G. Monni et al., 'The prevention of thalassemia in Sardinia'. *Clinical Genetics*, November 1989, 36 (5), 277–85, available from: https://pubmed.ncbi.nlm.nih.gov/2598483/. Also A. Cao, M. Furbetta, R. Galanello, M. A. Melis et al., 'Prevention of homozygous beta-thalassemia by carrier screening and prenatal diagnosis in Sardinia', *American Journal of Human Genetics*, July 1981, 33 (4), 592–605, available from: https://www.ncbi.nlm.nih.gov/pmc/articles/PMC1685095/.

3. See, for example, Virginia Bovell, 'Is There an Ethical Case for the Prevention and/or Cure of Autism?' in Hanna Bertilsdotter Rosqvist, Nick Chown and Anna Stenning (eds), *Neurodiversity Studies: A New Critical Paradigm*. London: Routledge (2020).

4. The multi-site autism research consortium AIMS-2-TRIALS offers the following distinction: 'AIMS-2-TRIALS does not aim to cure autism. We do aim to understand autism better and to test medical treatments that could alleviate specific difficulties that some autistic people experience'. (https://www.aims-2-trials.eu/about-aims-2-trials/ [accessed 25 September 2021]) Nonetheless, concerns about the underlying approach to genetic and other types of investigation

remain, regardless of how the goals are expressed. See, for example, the concerns about establishing large genetic databases, such as the proposed Spectrum 10K project: 'Whether Spectrum 10K, MSSNG, SPARK, and other massive databases become a footnote in historical scientific textbooks, possibly treating co-occurring conditions like seizures and GI issues, or leading to fetal autistic abortions is yet to be determined. Whatever the end result may be, many autistic people are justifiably worried given the evidence on the table.' Sebastian Rubino, 'Spectrum 10K: The Fallacy of Genetic Autism Studies', *TREMG*, 29 August 2021 (https://tremg.info/2021/08/29/spectrum-10k-the-fallacy-of-genetic-autism-studies/ [accessed 25 September 2021]).

5. Bethany Oakley, Julian Tillman, Jumana Ahmad, Daisy Crawley et al. (The EU-AIMS LEAP Group), 'How do core autism traits and associated symptoms relate to quality of life? Findings from the Longitudinal European Autism Project'. *Autism*, February 2021, 25 (2), 389–404. Article first published online 7 October 2020, available from: https://pubmed.ncbi.nlm.nih.gov/33023296/.

6. Sarah Cassidy, Louise Bradley, Rebecca Shaw and Simon Baron-Cohen, 'Risk markers for suicidality in autistic adults'. *Molecular Autism*, 2018, 9 (42), available from: https://doi.org/10.1186/s13229-018-0226-4. And S. A. Cassidy, K. Gould, E. Townsend, M. Pelton et al., 'Is Camouflaging Autistic Traits Associated with Suicidal Thoughts and Behaviours? Expanding the Interpersonal Psychological Theory of Suicide in an Undergraduate Student Sample'. *Journal of Autism and Developmental Disorders*, 2020, 50 (10), 3638–48, available from: https://doi.org/10.1007/s10803-019-04323-3.

36 SPRING AND SUMMER 2013

1. The press conference with Arsène Wenger, on the occasion of his visit to TreeHouse, televised by Sky Sports and described in

Chapter 25, was by far the most memorable of the various TV interviews I carried out during the campaigning years (with perhaps the exception of *The Wright Stuff*, in 2013, as retold in Chapter 28). During the campaigning years I also set foot twice in No. 10 Downing Street. The first occasion was in 1998, when I went with Nick to a reception for people of cultural and sporting significance. The second, surreal for being held one or two days before the Iraq War in March 2003, was a reception to celebrate excellence in special educational needs

2. Here I was referring to bioethical debates around antenatal selection against disability, and the notion of 'procreative beneficence' as advocated by John Harris – in *Enhancing Evolution: The Ethical Case for Making Better People*. Princeton, NJ: Princeton University Press (2007) – and Julian Savulescu, to whom I was referring in my journal. He wrote: 'Couples should employ genetic tests to have the child, *of the possible children they could have*, who will have the best opportunity of having the best life (subject to cost constraints).' ('Deaf Lesbians, "Designer Disability", and the Future of Medicine', p. 771, my italics).

3. For the importance of Person-Centred Planning in the transition process, see https://www.challengingbehaviour.org.uk/information-and-guidance/person-centred-support/transition-planning/ [accessed 25 September 2021].

37 Crisis

1. See the hard-hitting report published by the learning disability charity FitzRoy, *'Who will care after I'm gone?' An Insight into the Pressures Facing Parents of People with Learning Disabilities*. Petersfield: FitzRoy (2015).

38 Disagreements and The Empathy Question

1. Simon Baron-Cohen, *Zero Degrees of Empathy: A New Theory of Human Cruelty*. London: Penguin Books (2011).

2. Damian E.M. Milton, 'On the ontological status of autism: The double empathy problem'. *Disability and Society*, 2012, 27 (6), 883–7.

3. Timothy Krahn and Andrew Fenton, 'Autism, Empathy and Questions of Moral Agency'. *Journal for the Theory of Social Behaviour*, 2009, 39 (2), 145–66.

4. Alicia Lile, 'What I need and want', originally posted on the blog *Moonlit Lily*, 2011, available from: https://autisticadvo-cacy.org/2011/12/what-i-need-and-want/.

5. *Snow Cake*, Marc Evans, dir. (Revolution Films, 2006). You can hear Ros talking with Sigourney in an interview hosted by Uniquely Human: The Podcast, available from: https://uniquelyhuman.libsyn.com/special-release-logically-illogical-an-interview-with-ros-blackburn-with-special-guest-sigourney-weaver.

6. Conference referred to in: Elizabeth Pellicano and Marc Stears, 'Bridging autism, science and society: moving toward an ethically informed approach to autism research'. *Autism Research*, 2011, 4 (4), 271–82. First published 12 May 2011, available from: https://onlinelibrary.wiley.com/doi/10.1002/aur.201.

7. The conference was Autism Europe's 11th International Congress, which took place in Edinburgh on 16–18 September 2016. See https://www.autismeurope.org/latest-congress/. I shared the platform with Jonathan Green (child psychiatrist and Professor of Child and Adolescent Psychiatry at the University of Manchester), Martijn Dekker (originator of 'InLv', referred to in Chapter 3) and Damian Milton (who, as mentioned earlier in this chapter, begat the important observation that neurotypicals and autistics suffer from a mutual and reciprocal empathy prob-lem). Ros joined the panel via an online connection. Ros had to participate online because all attempts to find some-one to support her there in person had failed.

8. See the discussion on empathy at the start of this chapter.
9. See note 5 in chapter 2, p. 262.
10. By Deborah Barnbaum, for instance – see Chapter 31.

39 THE FUTURE OF AUTISM

1. Read more about the Spectrum 10K consultation in Louis Mylne, 'Summary of the Spectrum 10K Consultation (2021–2023)'. *Hopkins Van Mil*, 7 August 2023. [Online], available from: http://www.hopkinsvanmil.co.uk/news/ 2023/8/7/summary-of-the-spectrum-10k-consultation- 2021-2023. See also note 2, in Chapter 35.

2. DSM-5: American Psychiatric Association, *Diagnostic and Statistical Manual of Mental Disorders*. (5th edn) Washington, DC: APA (2013).

3. Laurent Mottron has used the distinction between proto-typical and syndromic autism to suggest that Early Intensive Behavioural Intervention (EIBI) is not useful for the former: 'Should we change targets and methods of early intervention in autism, in favor of a strengths-based education?'. *European Child & Adolescent Psychiatry*, 2017, 26(7), 815–25, available from: https://pubmed.ncbi.nlm. nih.gov/28181042/.

4. See C. Lord, T. Charman, A. Havdahl, P. Carbone et al., 'The *Lancet* Commission on the future of care and clinical research in autism'. *The Lancet*, 15 January 2022, 399 (10321), 271–334, available from: https://doi.org/10.1016/ S0140-6736(21)01541-5.

5. See, for example, Alison Singer, 'It's time to embrace "profound autism"'. *Spectrum*, 27 October 2022, available from: https://www.spectrumnews.org/opinion/viewpoint/ its-time-to-embrace-profound-autism/; versus Ashley Muskett, 'Response to The Idea of "Profound" Autism', *Ashley Muskett* [Personal Blog], 31 October 2022, available from: https://aemuskett.wixsite.com/ashleymuskett/post/

it-is-time-to-embrace-profound-autism-just-not-the-way-singer-thinks.

6. Ginny Russell, William Mandy, Daisy Elliott, Rhianna White et al., 'Selection bias on intellectual ability in autism research: a cross-sectional review and meta-analysis'. *Molecular Autism*, 2019, 10 (9), available from: https://doi.org/10.1186/s13229-019-0260-x.

7. Jonathan Green, 'Neurodiversity, autism, and health care'. *Child and Adolescent Mental Health*, 2023, 28 (3), 438–42, available from: https://doi.org/10.1111/camh.12663; and Jonathan Green, 'Autism as emergent and transactional'. *Frontiers in Psychiatry*, 2022, 13, available from: https://doi.org/10.3389/fpsyt.2022.988755.

8. Laura Dattaro, '"A catalyst for change": NIH makes first call for research supporting minimally verbal autistic people'. *Spectrum*, 18 July 2023, available from: https://www.spectrumnews.org/news/a-catalyst-for-change-nih-makes-first-call-for-research-supporting-minimally-verbal-autistic-people/.

9. To my knowledge, the first of these reports dates back to 2004, following a UK initiative instigated jointly by PACE and the NAS: Tony Charman and Pippa Clare, *Mapping autism research: Identifying UK priorities for the future*. London: National Autistic Society (2004). Its principal author, Tony Charman, went on to become one of the 'Big Names' cited towards the end of this book.

10. Green, 'Neurodiversity, autism, and health care'.

11. Robert Chapman and Virginia Bovell, 'Neurodiversity, Advocacy, Anti-Therapy', in P. Sturmey and J. Matson (eds), *Handbook of Autism and Pervasive Developmental Disorder*. New York: Springer (2022).

12. Samantha Easter and Amy S.F. Lutz, 'Building bridges: Collaboration across the autism community'. *Spectrum*, 24 October 2023, available from: https://www.spectrumnews.

org/opinion/viewpoint/building-bridges-collaboration-across-the-autism-community/?utm_source=Spectrum+Newsletters&utm_campaign=454f3ff117-DAILY+20231024+TUESDAY+%28BRIDGES%29&utm_medium=email&utm_term=0_529db1161f-454f3ff117-168640661.

13. Dinah Murray, Damian Milton, Jonathan Green and Jo Bervoets, 'The Human Spectrum: A Phenomenological Enquiry within Neurodiversity'. *Psychopathology*, 2023, 56 (3), 220–30, available from: https://doi.org/10.1159/000526213.

14. BBC News, 'Cawston Park: Vulnerable patient deaths prompt hospitals warning'. 9 September 2021. [Online], available from: https://www.bbc.co.uk/news/uk-england-norfolk-58466839.

15. Green, 'Neurodiversity, autism, and health care'.

40 VALUING LEARNING DISABILITY

1. Virginia Bovell, *Is the Prevention and/or Cure of Autism a Morally Legitimate Quest?* 2015. [PhD thesis]. University of Oxford. p. 299, available from: https://ora.ox.ac.uk/objects/uuid:59b5a983-b6a9-4f39-a7fd-0c67757aab73.

2. Theresa May, UK Prime Minister, used this phrase in 2017 to justify withholding pay increases to NHS staff. See Lizzie Dearden, 'Theresa May prompts anger after telling nurse who hasn't had pay rise for eight years: "There's no magic money tree"'. *Independent*, 3 June 2017, available from: https://www.independent.co.uk/news/uk/politics/theresa-may-nurse-magic-money-tree-bbcqt-question-time-pay-rise-eight-years-election-latest-a7770576.html.

3. See note 6 in Chapter 35, p. 278

4. Eva Feder Kittay, *Love's Labor: Essays on Women, Equality and Dependency*. New York; London: Routledge (1999), p. 173.

41 How Things Are Now

1. See, for example, the post 'On Autism', 20 July 2019, on Fergus's website, available from: https://oolong.co.uk/on-autism. See also http://monotropism.org which houses an archive of Dinah's work, as well as some of Fergus's work, and http://weirdpride.day which Fergus started partly as a tribute to her.

2. Ingmar Persson and Julian Savulescu, *Unfit for the Future: The Need for Moral Enhancement*. Oxford: Oxford University Press (2012).

Select Bibliography

Adams, Tim. 'Chris Packham: "People like me have a very aggravated sense of injustice"'. *Guardian*, 18 July 2021. [Online]. Available from https://www.theguardian.com/food/2021/jul/18/chris-packham-people-like-me-sense-of-injustice-autism-extinction-rebellion.

Adult recently diagnosed with autism spectrum disorder. [Question on social question-and-answer website]. *Quora*, 5 January 2022.

AIMS-2-TRIALS [Online]. https://www.aims-2-trials.eu/about-aims-2-trials/ [accessed 25 September 2021].

All Party Parliamentary Group on Autism. *Autism and education in England 2017: A report by the All Party Parliamentary Group on Autism on how the education system in England works for children and young people on the autism spectrum.* pdf [accessed 26 August 2021].

American Psychiatric Association. *Diagnostic and Statistical Manual of Mental Disorders.* (4th edn.) Washington, DC: APA (2000).

American Psychiatric Association. *Diagnostic and Statistical Manual of Mental Disorders.* (5th edn.) Washington, DC: APA (2013).

Andari, Elissar, Duhamel, Jean-René, Zalla, Tiziana, Herbrecht, Evelyn, Leboyer, Marion and Sirigu, Angela. 'Promoting social behaviour with oxytocin in high-functioning autism spectrum disorders'. *Proceedings of the National Academy of Sciences of the United States of America*, 2010, 107 (9), pp. 4,389–94.

ASAN. 'ASAN Commends FDA's Move to Appeal Judge Rotenberg Center Ruling'. 10 September 2021. [Online]. Available from: https://autisticadvocacy.org/2021/09/asan-commends-fdas-move-to-appeal-judge-rotenberg-center-ruling/.

ASAN. Symposium on Ethical, Legal and Social Implications of Autism Research. Held on 10 December 2011. [Online video of proceedings]. Available from: https://www.youtube.com/user/autselfadvocacyntwk.

Autism-Europe. 'XI Autism-Europe International Congress, Edinburgh, Scotland, 2016'. [Online]. https://www.autismeurope.org/latest-congress/.

Baeza-Velasco, Carolina, Cohen, David, Hamonet, Claude, Vlamynck, Elodie et al. 'Autism, Joint Hypermobility-Related Disorders and Pain'. *Frontiers in Psychiatry*, 7 December 2019, 9, Article 656. Available from: https://doi.org/10.3389/fpsyt.2018.00656.

Baggs, Amanda M. *In My Language*. 2007. [Online video]. Available from: https://www.youtube.com/watch?v=JnylM1hI2jc.

Bannow, Tara. 'Parents and clinicians say private equity's profit fixation is short-changing kids with autism'. *STAT*, 15 August 2022. [Online]. Available from: https://www.statnews.com/2022/08/15/private-equity-autism-aba-therapy/?utm_source=Spectrum+Newsletters&utm_campaign=d8ceb25035-EMAIL_CAMPAIGN_DAILY_20220816_TUESDAY&utm_medium=email&utm_term=0_529db1161f-d8ceb25035-168640661.

Barnbaum, Deborah R. *The Ethics of Autism: Among Them, but Not of Them*. Bloomington: Indiana University Press (2008).

Baron, Saskia. 'Autism unpacked: how my brother's autism has changed over 50 years and how the definition of autism as a whole has changed over his lifetime'. [Presentation]. Delivered at NAS Professional Conference, held on 5–6 March 2013, Harrogate.

Baron-Cohen, Simon. *Autism and Asperger syndrome: The Facts.* Oxford: OUP (2008).

Baron-Cohen, Simon. *The Essential Difference: Men, Women and the Extreme Male Brain.* London: Penguin (2004).

Baron-Cohen, Simon. *Zero Degrees of Empathy: A New Theory of Human Cruelty.* London: Penguin Books (2011).

BBC 1. *Paddy and Christine McGuinness: Our Family and Autism.* Lucy Wilcox, dir. (BBC1, 2021).

BBC 2. *Chris Packham: Asperger's and Me.* Charlie Russell, dir. (BBC2, 2017 and last aired on 3 March 2021). https://www.bbc.co.uk/programmes/b09b1zbb?.

BBC News. 'Autism and anxiety: One man "failed by the system"'. 27 August 2021. [Online]. Available from: https://www.bbc.co.uk/news/av/uk-58334061.

BBC News. 'Cawston Park: Vulnerable patient deaths prompt hospitals warning'. 9 September 2021. [Online]. Available from: https://www.bbc.co.uk/news/uk-england-norfolk-58466839.

BBC News. 'Down's syndrome: Abortion case heads to High Court'. 5 May 2021. [Online]. Available from: https://www.bbc.co.uk/news/uk-england-56982646.

Bettelheim, Bruno. *The Empty Fortress: Infantile Autism and the Birth of the Self.* New York: Free Press/Collier-Macmillan (1967).

Boait, Fran. 'The Truth Behind the "Magic Money Tree"'. *Positive Money*, n.d. [Online]. Available from: https://positivemoney.org/2017/06/magic-money-tree/.

Boseley, Sarah. 'Doctors turn on each other as MMR debate rages again: Architects of autism study embroiled in bitter dispute'. *Guardian*, 1 November 2003. Available from: https://www.theguardian.com/society/2003/nov/01/highereducation.medicineandhealth.

Bovell, Virginia. 'Campaigning for Autism Services: Reflections on the past, dreams for the future'. [Presentation]. Delivered on 12 January 2012 at the Autism Spectrum Disorder: from clinical practice to educational provision conference, held on 12–13 January 2012 at the Irish Centre for Autism and Neurodevelopmental Research, National University of Ireland, Galway.

Bovell, Virginia. *Is the Prevention and/or Cure of Autism a Morally Legitimate Quest?* 2015. [PhD thesis]. University of Oxford. Available from: https://ora.ox.ac.uk/objects/uuid:59b5a983-b6a9-4f39-a7fd-0c67757aab73.

Bovell, Virginia. 'Is There an Ethical Case for the Prevention and/or Cure of Autism?' in Hanna Bertilsdotter Rosqvist, Nick Chown and Anna Stenning (eds), *Neurodiversity Studies: A New Critical Paradigm*. London: Routledge (2020).

Broach, Steve and Clements, Luke. *Disabled Children: A Legal Handbook*. (3rd edn) London: Legal Action Group (2020).

Buchanan, Allen, Brock, Dan W., Daniels, Norman and Wikler, Daniel. *From Chance to Choice: Genetics & Justice*. New York, Cambridge: Cambridge University Press (2000).

Bunting, Madeleine. *Labours of Love: The Crisis of Care*. London: Granta (2020).

Cao, A., Furbetta, M., Galanello, R., Melis, M. A. et al. 'Prevention of homozygous beta-thalassemia by carrier screening and prenatal diagnosis in Sardinia'. *American Journal of Human Genetics*, July 1981, 33 (4), 592–605. Available from: https://www.ncbi.nlm.nih.gov/pmc/articles/PMC1685095/.

Cao, A., Rosatelli, C., Galanello, R., Monni, G. et al. 'The prevention of thalassemia in Sardinia'. *Clinical Genetics*, November 1989, 36 (5), 277–85. Available from: https://pubmed.ncbi.nlm.nih.gov/2598483/.

Carey, Matt. 'Scientists must curb tendency to try untested treatments'. *Spectrum*, 12 May 2016. [Online]. Available from: https://www.spectrumnews.org/opinion/viewpoint/scientists–must–curb-tendency-to-try-untested-treatments/.

Carlson, Doreen. [Letter to the editor]. *Independent*, 14 November 2007.

Carlson, Licia. *The Faces of Intellectual Disability: Philosophical Reflections*. Bloomington: Indiana University Press (2010).

Cassidy, Sarah, Bradley, Louise, Shaw, Rebecca and Baron-Cohen, Simon. 'Risk markers for suicidality in autistic adults'. *Molecular Autism*, 2018, 9 (42). Available from: https://doi.org/10.1186/s13229-018-0226-4.

Cassidy, S.A., Gould, K., Townsend, E., Pelton, M., Robertson, A.E. and Rodgers, J. 'Is Camouflaging Autistic Traits Associated with Suicidal Thoughts and Behaviours? Expanding the Interpersonal Psychological Theory of Suicide in an Undergraduate Student Sample'. *Journal of Autism and Developmental Disorders*, 2020, 50 (10), 3638–48. Available from: https://doi.org/10.1007/s10803-019-04323-3.

Challenging Behaviour Foundation. 'Transition planning'. n.d. [Online]. Available from: https://www.challengingbehaviour.org.uk/information-and-guidance/person-centred-support/transition-planning/.

Chapman, Matthew. 'Asperger's abuse inquiry pledged'. 25 September 2004. [Online]. Available from: http://news.bbc.co.uk/1/hi/health/3687612.stm.

Chapman, Matthew. 'Bestseller helps parents fight accusations of child abuse: Novel has shed light on Asperger's Syndrome but families still find themselves under investigation'. *Guardian*, 26 September 2004. Available from: https://www.theguardian.com/society/2004/sep/26/childrensservices.books.

Chapman, Robert and Bovell, Virginia. 'Neurodiversity, Advocacy, Anti-Therapy', in P. Sturmey and J. Matson (eds), *Handbook of Autism and Pervasive Developmental Disorder*. New York: Springer (2022).

Charman, Tony and Clare, Pippa. *Mapping autism research: Identifying UK priorities for the future.* London: National Autistic Society (2004).

Chrisafis, Angelique. 'Despair of mother in fatal leap with son'. *Guardian*, 30 January 2002. Available from: https://www.theguardian.com/uk/2002/jan/30/angeliquechrisafis.

Claiborne Park, Clara. *The Siege.* New York: Harcourt, Brace & World (1967).

Collins, Paul. *Not Even Wrong: A Father's Journey into the Lost History of Autism.* New York: Bloomsbury Publishing (2004).

Communication Matters. 'What is AAC?'. n.d. [Online]. Available from: https://www.communicationmatters.org.uk/what-is-aac/.

Culmer, Phil. [Letter to the editor]. *Independent*, 10 November 2007.

Dattaro, Laura. '"A catalyst for change": NIH makes first call for research supporting minimally verbal autistic people'. *Spectrum*, 18 July 2023. [Online]. Available from: https://www.spectrumnews.org/news/a-catalyst-for-change-nih-makes-first-call-for-research-supporting-minimally-verbal-autistic-people/.

Dawson, Michelle. 'Challenges to autism intervention research: costs, benefits, problems and solutions'. [Keynote speech.] Delivered on 28 February 2012 at the National Autistic Society Professional Conference – Working Together for Better Outcomes, held on 28–29 February 2012, Manchester.

Dawson, Michelle. 'The Misbehaviour of Behaviourists: Ethical Challenges to the Autism–ABA Industry'. 2004. [Online]. Available from: http://www.sentex.ca/~nexus23/naa_aba.html.

Dawson, Michelle. 'Oxytocin versus autism: A cure for altruism'. 17 February 2010. [Online]. Available from: http://autismcrisis.blogspot.co.uk/2010/02/oxytocin-versus-autism-cure-for.html.

Dearden, Lizzie. 'Theresa May prompts anger after telling nurse who hasn't had pay rise for eight years: "There's no magic money tree"'. *Independent*, 3 June 2017. Available from: https://www.independent.co.uk/news/uk/politics/theresa-may-nurse-magic-money-tree-bbcqt-question-time-pay-rise-eight-years-election-latest-a7770576.html.

Diament, Michelle. 'Autism Speaks No Longer Seeking Cure'. *Disability Scoop*, 14 October 2016. [Online]. Available from: https://www.disabilityscoop.com/2016/10/14/autism-speaks-no-longer-cure/22884/.

Drake, Haywood. [Letter to the editor]. *Independent*, 14 November 2007.

Eisenstein, Michael. 'Gene therapies close in on a cure for sickle-cell disease'. *Nature*, 25 August 2021. Available from: https://www.nature.com/articles/d41586-021-02138-w [accessed 25 September 2021].

Easter, Samantha and Lutz, Amy S. F. 'Building bridges: Collaboration across the autism community'. *Spectrum*, 24 October 2023. [Online]. Available from: https://www.spectrumnews.org/opinion/viewpoint/building-bridges-collaboration-across-the-autism-community/?utm_source=Spectrum+Newsletters&utm_campaign=454f3ff117-DAILY+20231024+TUESDAY+%28BRIDGES%29&utm_medium=email&utm_term=0_529db1161f-454f3ff117-168640661.

Elliott, Angie. [Letter to the editor]. *Independent*, 22 November 2007.

Feinberg, Joel. 'The Child's Right to an Open Future', in William Aiken and Hugh LaFollette (eds), *Whose Child? Children's Rights, Parental Authority, and State Power*. Totowa, NJ: Rowman and Littlefield (1980), 124–53.

Feinstein, Adam. *A History of Autism: Conversations with the Pioneers*. Chichester: Wiley-Blackwell (2010).

Fitzpatrick, Michael. *Defeating Autism: A Damaging Delusion*. Abingdon: Routledge (2009).

FitzRoy. *'Who will care after I'm gone?' An Insight into the Pressures Facing Parents of People with Learning Disabilities.* Petersfield: FitzRoy (2015).

Fletcher-Watson, Sue and Happé, Francesca. *Autism: A New Introduction to Psychological Theory and Current Debate.* Abingdon: Routledge (2019).

Forrest, Celia. [Letter to the editor]. *Independent,* 10 November 2007.

Frith, Uta. *Autism: Explaining the Enigma.* (2nd edn) Oxford: Blackwell (2003).

Gillberg, Christopher. 'Response to Mottron'. *Autism Research,* 14 (10), 2228–9. First published 2 June 2021. Available from: https://doi.org/10.1002/aur.2547 [accessed 29 September 2021].

Glover, Jonathan. *Choosing Children: Genes, Disability, and Design.* Oxford: Oxford University Press (2006).

Grandin, Temple. *Thinking in Pictures: My Life with Autism.* (Expanded edition) New York: Vintage (2006).

Great Britain. Autism Act 2009. London: The Stationery Office. Available from: https://www.legislation.gov.uk/ukpga/2009/15/contents.

Great Britain. Equality Act 2010. London: The Stationery Office. Available from: http://legislation.gov.uk/ukpga/2010/15/contents.

Green, Jonathan. 'Autism as emergent and transactional'. *Frontiers in Psychiatry,* 2022, 13. Available from: https://doi.org/10.3389/fpsyt.2022.988755.

Green, Jonathan. 'Neurodiversity, autism, and health care'. *Child and Adolescent Mental Health,* 2023, 28 (3), 438–42. Available from: https://doi.org/10.1111/camh.12663.

Grinker, Roy Richard. *Isabel's World: Autism and the Making of a Modern Epidemic.* London: Icon Books (2009).

Groove Armada. 'If Everybody Looked the Same', in *Vertigo.* Jive 0530332 (1999). [CD].

Harris, John. *Enhancing Evolution: The Ethical Case for Making Better People*. Princeton, NJ: Princeton University Press (2007).

Heslop, Pauline, Blair, Peter, Fleming, Peter, Hoghton, Matt et al. *Confidential Inquiry into premature deaths of people with learning disabilities (CIPOLD)*. Norah Fry Research Centre: Bristol (2013). Available from: https://www.bristol.ac.uk/media-library/sites/cipold/migrated/documents/fullfinalreport.pdf.

Holm, Søren. 'Ethical Issues in Pre-implantation Diagnosis', in John Harris and Søren Holm (eds), *The Future of Human Reproduction: Ethics, Choice and Regulation*. Oxford: Clarendon Press (1998), 176–90.

Hornby, Nick. 'Life with Danny'. *Daily Telegraph Weekend*, 6 December 1997.

Hornby, Nick (ed.). *Speaking with the Angel*. Harmondsworth: Penguin Books (2000).

Hornby, Nick. *31 Songs*. London: Penguin (2003).

Iemmi, Valentina, Knapp, Martin and Ragan, Ian on behalf of the National Autism Project. *The Autism Dividend: Reaping the rewards of better investment*. London: London School of Economics and Political Science (2017).

Izuma, Keise, Matsumoto, Kenji, Camerer, Colin F. and Adolphs, Ralph. 'Insensitivity to social reputation in autism'. *Proceedings of the National Academy of Sciences*, 10 October 2011, 108 (42), 17302–7. Available from: http://www.pnas.org/content/108/42/17302.full.

Jardine, Cassandra. 'Should we want to cure autism?'. *Telegraph*, 22 October 2008.

Jarrett, Simon. 'Editor's Diary: Outfoxed by morality'. *Community Living*, 2021, 34 (2), p. 25.

Jarrett, Simon. *Those They Called Idiots: The Idea of the Disabled Mind from 1700 to the Present Day*. London: Reaktion Books (2020).

Jordan, Rita, Jones, Glenys and Murray, Dinah. *Educational Interventions for Children with Autism: A Literature Review of*

Recent and Current Research (DfEE Research Report No. 77). London: DfEE (1998).

Kapp, Steven K. (ed.). *Autistic Community and the Neurodiversity Movement: Stories from the Frontline*. Singapore: Springer Nature (2020).

Kapp, Steven K., Steward, Robyn, Crane, Laura, Elliott, Daisy et al. '"People should be allowed to do what they like": Autistic adults' views and experiences of stimming'. *Autism*, 2019, 23 (7), 1782–92. Available from: https://doi.org/10.1177/1362361319829628.

Keeler, Helen. 'Unnatural selection'. *BioNews*, 538, 14 December 2009. Available from: https://www.bionews.org.uk/page_92061.

Keer, Matt. '95% of decisions in favour of parents, but nobody wins at the SEND Tribunal'. *Special Needs Jungle*, 11 December 2020. [Online]. Available from: https://www.specialneedsjungle.com/95-decisions-favour-parents-nobody-wins-send-tribunal/ [accessed 26 August 2021].

Kirby, Megan S., Spencer, Trina D. and Spiker, Shane T. 'Humble Behaviorism Redux'. *Behavior and Social Issues*, 2022. Available from: https://doi.org/10.1007/s42822-022-00092-4.

Kittay, Eva Feder. *Love's Labor: Essays on Women, Equality and Dependency*. New York; London: Routledge (1999).

Krahn, Timothy and Fenton, Andrew. 'Autism, Empathy and Questions of Moral Agency'. *Journal for the Theory of Social Behaviour*, 2009, 39 (2), 145–66.

Kupferstein, Henny. 'Evidence of increased PTSD symptoms in autistics exposed to applied behavior analysis'. *Advances in Autism*, 2018, 4 (1), 19–29.

Laurance, Jeremy. 'Autism: What are the ethics of treating disability? A row about the correct response to the condition – acceptance or treatment – is dividing campaigners and carers'. *Independent*, 16 November 2007.

Lawson, Wendy. *Concepts of Normality: The Autistic and Typical Spectrum*. London: Jessica Kingsley Publishers (2008).

Lawson, Wendy. *Life Behind Glass: A Personal Account of Autism Spectrum Disorder*. London: Jessica Kingsley Publishers (2001).

Lehrer, R. *Golem Girl: A Memoir*. London: Virago Press (2021).

Lile, Alicia. 'What I need and want', originally posted on the blog *Moonlit Lily*, 2011. Available from: https://autisticadvocacy.org/2011/12/what-i-need-and-want/.

Lord, C., Charman, T., Havdahl, A., Carbone, P. et al. 'The *Lancet* Commission on the future of care and clinical research in autism'. *The Lancet*, 15 January 2022, 399 (10321), 271–334. Available from: https://doi.org/10.1016/S0140-6736(21)01541-5.

Lovaas, O. Ivar. 'Behavioral treatment and normal educational and intellectual functioning in young autistic children'. *Journal of Consulting and Clinical Psychology*, 1987, 55, 3–9.

Maddrell, Geoffrey. [Letter to the editor]. *Independent*, 10 November 2007.

Maenner, M. J., Warren, Z., Williams, A. R., Amoakohene, E. et al. 'Prevalence and Characteristics of Autism Spectrum Disorder Among Children Aged 8 Years – Autism and Developmental Disabilities Monitoring Network, 11 Sites, United States, 2020'. *MMWR Surveillance Summaries*, 2023, 72 (2), 1–14. Available from: http://dx.doi.org/10.15585/mmwr.ss7202a1.

Mason, Micheline. *Incurably Human*. (2nd edn) Nottingham: Inclusive Solutions (2005).

Maurice, Catherine. *Let Me Hear Your Voice: A Family's Triumph Over Autism*. New York: Random House (1993).

McEachin, John J., Smith, Tristram and Lovaas, O. Ivar. 'Long-Term Outcome for Children with Autism Who Received Early Intensive Behavioral Treatment'. *American Journal on Mental Retardation*, 1993, 97 (4), 359–72.

McGill, Owen and Robinson, Anna. '"Recalling hidden harms":
    autistic experiences of childhood applied behavioural anal-
    ysis (ABA)'. *Advances in Autism*, 2021, 7 (4), 269–82. Available
    from: https://doi.org/10.1108/AIA-04-2020-0025.

McGuinness, Christine. *Christine McGuinness: A Beautiful
    Nightmare*. London: Mirror Books (2021).

McMahan, Jeff. *The Ethics of Killing*. New York: Oxford
    University Press (2003).

Middleton, Benet. [Letter to the editor]. *Independent*, 10
    November 2007.

Milton, Damian E. M. 'On the ontological status of autism: The
    double empathy problem'. *Disability and Society*, 2012, 27
    (6), 883–7.

Moore, Charlotte. *George and Sam*. London: Penguin Books
    (2012).

Mottron, Laurent. 'Should we change targets and methods of
    early intervention in autism, in favor of a strengths-based
    education?' *European Child & Adolescent Psychiatry*, 2017, 26,
    815–25. Available from: https://link.springer.com/article/
    10.1007%2Fs00787-017-0955-55.

Murray, Dinah. 'Autistic People Against Neuroleptic Abuse', in
    Steven K. Kapp (ed.), *Autistic Community and the Neurodiversity
    Movement: Stories from the Frontline*. Singapore: Springer
    Nature (2020), 51–63.

Murray, Dinah. 'From Protest to Taskforce', in Steven K. Kapp
    (ed.), *Autistic Community and the Neurodiversity Movement:
    Stories from the Frontline*. Singapore: Springer Nature (2020),
    277–85.

Murray, Dinah, Lesser, Mike and Lawson, Wendy. 'Attention,
    monotropism and the diagnostic criteria for autism'. *Autism*,
    2005, 9 (2), 136–56.

Murray, Dinah, Milton, Damian, Green, Jonathan and Bervoets,
    Jo. 'The Human Spectrum: A Phenomenological Enquiry
    within Neurodiversity'. *Psychopathology*, 2023, 56 (3),

220–30. Available from: https://doi.org/10.1159/00052 6213.

Murray, Fergus. 'On Autism'. 20 July 2019. [Online]. Available from: https://oolong.co.uk/on-autism.

Muskett, Ashley. 'Response to The Idea of "Profound" Autism'. *Ashley Muskett* [Personal Blog], 31 October 2022. Available from: https://aemuskett.wixsite.com/ashleymuskett/post/ it-is-time-to-embrace-profound-autism-just-not-the-way-singer-thinks.

Mylne, Louis. 'Summary of the Spectrum 10K Consultation (2021–2023)'. *Hopkins Van Mil*, 7 August 2023. [Online]. Available from: http://www.hopkinsvanmil.co.uk/news/ 2023/8/7/summary-of-the-spectrum-10k-consultation-2021-2023.

Ne'eman, Ari. *The Right to Live in This World: The Untold Story of Disability in America.* New York: Simon & Schuster (2021).

NeuroClastic. '900 ABA Professionals Have Weighed in on the Use of Electroshock at Judge Rotenberg Center'. 26 August 2021. [Online]. Available from: https://neuroclastic. com/900-aba-professionals-have-weighed-in-on-the-use-of-electroshock-at-judge-rotenberg-cennter/.

NHS. 'Overview – Fabricated or induced illness'. [Online]. Available from: https://www.nhs.uk/mental-health/condi-tions/fabricated-or-induced-illness/overview/.

NHS Commissioning Board. *Clinical Commissioning Policy: Pre-implantation Genetic Diagnosis (PGD).* April 2013. Available from: https://www.england.nhs.uk/wp-content/ uploads/2013/04/e01-p-a.pdf.

NICE. 'Autism: The management and support of children and young people on the autism spectrum'. (NICE clinical guideline 170). London: NICE (2013).

Nicolle, Lauren. 'Thousands of Children with SEND unable to access formal education'. *Learning Disability Today*, 14 February 2024. Available from: https://www.learningdis

abilitytoday.co.uk/news/thousands-of-children-with-send-unable-to-access-formal-education/.

Oakley, Bethany, Tillman, Julian, Ahmad, Jumana, Crawley, Daisy et al. (The EU-AIMS LEAP Group). 'How do core autism traits and associated symptoms relate to quality of life? Findings from the Longitudinal European Autism Project'. *Autism*, February 2021, 25 (2), 389–404. Article first published online 7 October 2020. Available from: https://journals.sagepub.com/doi/10.1177/1362361320959959.

Office of Autism Research Coordination. NIH-IACC Workshop: Ethical, Legal and Social Implications of Autism Research (ELSI). Held on 26 September–1 October 2011. [Online videocast]. Available from: http://nih.granicus.com/MediaPlayer.php?view_id=7&clip_id=367.

Offit, Paul A. *Autism's False Prophets: Bad Science, Risky Medicine, and the Search for a Cure*. New York: Columbia University Press (2008).

Pellicano, Elizabeth, Dinsmore, Adam and Charman, Tony. *A Future Made Together: Shaping Autism Research in the UK*. London: Institute of Education (2013).

Pellicano, Elizabeth and Stears, Marc. 'Bridging autism, science and society: moving toward an ethically informed approach to autism research'. *Autism Research*, 2011, 4 (4), 271–82. First published 12 May 2011. Available from: https://onlinelibrary.wiley.com/doi/10.1002/aur.201.

Persson, Ingmar and Savulescu, Julian. *Unfit for the Future: The Need for Moral Enhancement*. Oxford: Oxford University Press (2012).

Pickles, Andrew, Le Couteur, Ann, Leadbitter, Kathy, Salomone, Erica et al. 'Parent-mediated social communication therapy for young children with autism (PACT): long-term follow-up of a randomised controlled trial'. *The Lancet*, 19 November 2016, 388 (10059), 2501–9.

Available from: https://doi.org/10.1016/S0140-6736(16) 31229-6.

Quarmby, Katharine. *Scapegoat: Why We Are Failing Disabled People*. London: Portobello Books (2011).

Rimland, Bernard. *Infantile Autism: The Syndrome and Its Implications for a Neural Theory of Behavior*. New York: Appleton-Century-Crofts (1964).

Roman-Urrestarazu, Andres, Kessel, Robin van, Allison, Carrie, Matthews, Fiona E. et al. 'Association of Race/Ethnicity and Social Disadvantage With Autism Prevalence in 7 Million School Children in England'. *JAMA Pediatrics*, 2021, 175 (6), doi: 10.1001/jamapediatrics.2021.0054. Available from: https://jamanetwork.com/journals/jama-pediatrics/fullarticle/2777821.

Royal College of Physicians, Royal College of Pathologists and British Society for Genetic Medicine. *Ethical issues in prenatal genetic diagnosis: Guidance for clinical practice*. Report of the Joint Committee on Genomics in Medicine. London: RCP, RCPath and BSGM (2022). Available from: https://www.rcplondon.ac.uk/projects/outputs/ethical-issues-prenatal-genetic-diagnosis.

Rubino, Sebastian. 'Spectrum 10k: The Fallacy of Genetic Autism Studies'. *TREMG*, 29 August 2021. [Online]. Available from: https://tremg.info/2021/08/29/spectrum-10k-the-fallacy-of-genetic-autism-studies/ [accessed 25 September 2021].

Russell, Ginny, Mandy, William, Elliott, Daisy, White, Rhianna et al. 'Selection bias on intellectual ability in autism research: a cross-sectional review and meta-analysis'. *Molecular Autism*, 2019, 10 (9). Available from: https://doi.org/10.1186/s13229-019-0260-x.

Ryan, Sara. *Justice for Laughing Boy: Connor Sparrowhawk – A death by Indifference*. London: Jessica Kingsley Publishers (2018).

Salman, Saba (ed.). *Made Possible: Stories of success by people with learning disabilities – in their own words*. London: Unbound (2020).

Savulescu, Julian. 'Deaf Lesbians, "Designer Disability", and the Future of Medicine'. *British Medical Journal*, 2002, 325, 771–3.

Schreibman, Laura. *The Science and Fiction of Autism*. London: Harvard University Press (2005).

Scully, Jackie Leach. *Disability Bioethics: Moral Bodies, Moral Difference*. Plymouth: Rowman and Littlefield (2008).

Silberman, Steve. *NeuroTribes: The Legacy of Autism and How to Think Smarter About People Who Think Differently*. London: Allen & Unwin (2015).

Sinclair, Jim. 'Don't Mourn for Us'. Autism Network International newsletter *Our Voice*, 1993, 1 (3). [Online]. Available from: http://www.autreat.com/dont_mourn.html.

Singer, Alison. 'It's time to embrace "profound autism"'. *Spectrum*, 27 October 2022. [Online]. Available from: https://www. spectrumnews.org/opinion/viewpoint/its-time-to-embrace-profound-autism/.

Singer, Peter. *Animal Liberation*. London: Pimlico (1995).

Sirr, Steph. [Letter to the editor]. *Independent*, 17 November 2007.

Solomon, Andrew. *Far From the Tree: A Dozen Kinds of Love*. London: Chatto & Windus (2013).

Solomon, Andrew. *The Noonday Demon: An Atlas of Depression*. New York: Simon and Schuster (2001).

Something About Us. 2008. [Online video]. Available from: https://www.youtube.com/watch?v=J-014P0hQ6w (Part 1) and https://www.youtube.com/watch?v=Dna1 Z41_w3ca (Part 2).

Stanton, Mike. *Learning to Live with High Functioning Autism: A Parent's Guide for Professionals*. London: Jessica Kingsley Publishers (2000).

Starr, Sandy. 'How to talk about genome editing'. *British Medical Bulletin*, June 2018, 126 (1), 5–12. Available from: https://doi.org/10.1093/bmb/ldy015.

Starr, Sandy. Speech given at the Autism, Ethics and the Good Life conference held at the British Academy in London on 2 April 2012. Text available online from: https://www.spiked-online.com/2012/04/23/is-autism-just-another-identity/#.VCA4XJRdVvo.

Tapper, James. 'Fury at "do not resuscitate" notices given to Covid patients with learning disabilities'. *Observer*, 13 February 2021. Available from: https://www.theguardian.com/world/2021/feb/13/new-do-not-resuscitate-orders-imposed-on-covid-19-patients-with-learning-difficulties.

Thomas, R.S. 'Balance'. *Frequencies*. London: Macmillan (1978).

Timimi, Sami, Gardner, Neil and McCabe, Brian. *The Myth of Autism: Medicalising Men's Social and Emotional Competence*. Basingstoke: Palgrave Macmillan (2011).

Today. Discussion between Richard Mills and original author of Treating Autism letter to the *Independent*. BBC Radio 4. 2 November 2007. [Radio broadcast].

Treating Autism. [Letter to the editor]. *Independent*, 8 November 2007.

Union of the Physically Impaired Against Segregation. *Fundamental Principles of Disability*. London, UPIAS (1976).

Veverka, Yev. 'Applied behavior analysis and autism: Flawed application of a proven science'. *Spectrum*, 1 September 2022. [Online]. Available from: https://www.spectrumnews.org/opinion/viewpoint/applied-behavior-analysis-and-autism-flawed-application-of-a-proven-science/?utm_source=Spectrum+Newsletters&utm_campaign=a0dc552884-EMAIL_CAMPAIGN_DAILY_20220901&utm_medium=email&utm_term=0_529db1161f-a0dc552884-168640661.

302 DANNY'S PEOPLE

Wady, Paul. [Letter to the editor]. *Independent*, 14 November 2007.

Wakefield, Andrew, Murch, Simon, Anthony, Andrew, Walker-Smith, John et al. 'RETRACTED: Ileal-lymphoid-nodular hyperplasia, non-specific colitis, and pervasive developmental disorder in children'. *The Lancet*, 28 February 1998, 351 (9103), 637–41. Available from: https://www.thelancet.com/journals/lancet/article/PIIS0140-6736(97)11096-0/fulltext.

Waltz, Mitzi. 'The Production of the "Normal" Child: Neurodiversity and the Commodification of Parenting' in Hanna Rosqvist, Nick Chown, Anna Stenning (eds) *Neurodiversity Studies: A New Critical Paradigm*. Abingdon: Routledge (2020).

Wason, Armorer. *Constructive Campaigning for Autism Services: The PACE Parents' Handbook*. London: Jessica Kingsley Publishers (2005).

Wharmby, Pete. *Untypical: How the world isn't built for autistic people and what we should all do about it*. London: Mudlark/Harper Collins (2023).

Wilkinson, Stephen. *Choosing Tomorrow's Children: The Ethics of Selective Reproduction*. Oxford: Oxford University Press (2010).

Williams, Donna. *Nobody Nowhere: The Remarkable Autobiography of an Autistic Girl*. London: Jessica Kingsley Publishers (1998).

Wing, Lorna. *The Autistic Spectrum: A Guide for Parents and Professionals*. London: Constable & Robinson (1996).

Wolpert, Lewis. *Malignant Sadness: The Anatomy of Depression*. London: Faber and Faber (2001).

World Health Organization. *International Statistical Classification of Diseases and Related Health Problems*. Geneva: Author (2010).

Zhang, Sarah. 'The Last Children of Down Syndrome'. *The Atlantic*, December 2020. Available from: https://www.theatlantic.com/magazine/archive/2020/12/the-last-children-of-down-syndrome/616928/ [accessed 1 September 2021].

Ziegel, Sarah. *Marching to a Different Beat: A family's journey with autism*. London: Lapis Print (2022)

ACKNOWLEDGEMENTS

I am so grateful to all who have been part of Danny's and my life, who have helped shape my priorities and my beliefs, and who have taught me about loyalty and love. I don't know how Danny and I would have made it this far without you. Most of you are named in the book and as such I thank you all, from the bottom of my heart.

Caroline Dawnay and Kat Aitken at United Agents, Cecilia Stein and all the wonderful Oneworld people who believed that the book needed to see the light of day and who helped its evolution with such skill and understanding – it has been a complete joy, as well as a relief, to follow your guidance. I couldn't have wished for a nicer group of people to lead me to the finishing tape.

Among so many people who have been willing to engage in the battle of ideas, I would like in particular to thank Leneh Buckle, Robert Chapman, Tony Charman, Nick Chown, Simon Baron-Cohen, Laura Crane, Martijn Dekker, Louise Denne, Jonathan Green, Jane Lewis, Jane McCready, Damian Milton, Liz Pellicano, Sandy Starr and Andy Swartfigure. And there are many more – apologies for not mentioning you all by name. We haven't always agreed, of course, but the integrity and good will with which our discourse has been conducted is all-important. Any technical and conceptual errors in trying to outline the issues are entirely my own.

Sue Tyley – you are a complete star. Without you, the interminable process of writing would never have ended.

I also want to salute my friends and colleagues in Islington and beyond, as well as everyone – neurodivergent and neurotypical – who is engaged in the struggle to make the world a place that thrives through its diversity, and in which all kinds of people can have good lives. I learn from you every day.

Requiring particular thanks are:

• Elinor Pearce – the inspiration for her mother Clare Palmer's activism. It is Clare – herself a writer – who first suggested I write about some of the events in this book, and whose friendship and insights continue to nourish me.

• Everyone involved in the TreeHouse story – the children and their families, the teachers, the trustees, the supporters and helpers. *A luta continua* – we are all part of something bigger than ourselves as we endeavour to keep listening and learning.

• My neighbours who tolerated the decibels of Danny's distress, day and night, and who never complained.

• Nick Coleman – thank you not only for ploughing through a very early draft of *Danny's People* with the necessary tact and expertise, but also – with Jane Acton – for supplying the lifeline of dancing to brilliant music during the Rarely Groove years; for loyalty and hospitality; for steadfast friendship.

• Jonathan Glover and Pat Walsh, who provided an all-important grounding in medical ethics, and – long ago now – Petal O'Hea, who taught me that we should approach the field of economics with our hearts as well as our brains.

• Saskia Baron, Penny Bernstock, Laura Fleminger, Sally Griffin, Philip O'Hara, Pamela Reitemeier, Paula Sanchez and Anne Tyley – how lucky I have been that our paths have crossed, and that you were kind enough to give feedback on drafts of the book.

- My lifelong friends – in (I think) chronological order: Susie, Philis, Sarah, Lucinda, Fiona, Carol and Christine (x 2).

And thank you finally to my three sets of family – Bovells, Hornby/Harrises and Hedleys. Here I run out of words. You are just so dear to me. Where would I be without you?